DIAGNOSTIC PROBLEMS IN DERMATOLOGY

DIAGNOSTIC PROBLEMS IN DERMATOLOGY

NEIL H COX

BSc (HONS), FRCP
Consultant Dermatologist
Cumberland Infirmary
Carlisle, UK

CLIFFORD M LAWRENCE

MD, FRCP
Consultant Dermatologist
Royal Victoria Infirmary
Newcastle, UK

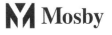 Mosby

London Philadelphia St. Louis Sydney Tokyo

Project Manager:	Peter Harrison
Development Editor:	Gina Almond
Designer:	Paul Phillips
Layout Artist:	Gisli Thor
Cover Design:	Paul Phillips
Production:	Hamish Adamson
Index:	Dr Laurence Errington
Publisher:	Richard Furn

Copyright © 1998 Mosby International Publishers Limited

Published in 1998 by Mosby, an imprint of Mosby International Publishers Limited

Printed by Grafos S.A. Arte sobre papel, Barcelona, Spain

ISBN 0 7234 2790 9

For full details of all Mosby titles, please write to Mosby International Publishers Limited, Lynton House, 7–12 Tavistock Square, London WC1H 9LB, England.

A CIP catalogue record for this book is available from the British Library.

Library of Congress Cataloging-in-Publication Data applied for.

Preface

This book is designed to help non-dermatologists to reach a differential diagnosis between disorders which are frequently confused with each other. Most of our choices are direct comparisons between two specific disorders, but some are between specific processes (e.g. scarring and non-scarring alopecias) where these distinctions have important implications. Likewise, most comparisons relate to common disorders whilst a few include uncommon but important differential diagnoses.

The book is organised into the body sites at which there may be difficulty differentiating between each pair of disorders, and each comparison is laid out as a double page spread for ease of access. Within each pair of disorders, the aim is to compare and contrast, with the emphasis on features which have discriminatory value;

other disorders which may enter the differential diagnosis are listed and illustrated, and extensive cross referencing is used to direct the reader to other forms or body sites of the same disorders.

Most of the illustrations that we have used are our own photographs, but a small number have been generously lent to us by colleagues, and these are acknowledged in the legends. We are particularly grateful for the support of our families during this project and take this opportunity to thank Fi, David and Kathy Cox, and Anne, Tom, Jo, Chris and James Lawrence for their patience and help.

NHC
CML

Contents

Contents

Psoriasis v. seborrhoeic dermatitis (adults)

Common presenting feature: scalp scaling with underlying erythema and a variable degree of itch.

Rationale for comparison: these two conditions are often confused but treatment options and prognosis differ.

Other differential diagnoses: tinea capitis (p. 8); discoid lupus erythematosus and other scarring alopecias (p. 6); scalp infestation; eczema affecting the scalp.

Conclusion and key points: recognizing the difference between these two disorders widens the treatment options beyond keratolytics, emollients, tar preparations and corticosteroids, all of which may be used for either (see 'Comparative features'). Silvery scale, and sharply demarcated lesions favour a diagnosis of psoriasis. When distant lesions are present, these are the most useful discriminators (especially psoriasis on limbs), but there may not be any lesions at other sites. In some patients with scalp involvement alone, it may be impossible to distinguish confidently between these two dermatoses.

Comparative features		
Disorder	**Scalp psoriasis**	**Scalp seborrhoeic dermatitis**
Age	Any	Any (childhood seborrhoeic dermatitis of scalp is rarely confused, and usually non-inflammatory)
Sex	Either	Either, more common in males
Family history	May be positive for psoriasis at any site	None
Sites	Any area of scalp, especially the forehead scalp margin, occiput, and above the ears, may be involved. Lesions are usually sharply localized.	Any area of scalp may be involved. This disorder is characteristically mild and diffuse in distribution on the scalp (when it is known as 'dandruff' or 'pityriasis capitis'). Diagnostic confusion may occur when lesions are more localized.
Symptoms	None, itch	
Signs common to both	A scaly scalp rash with underlying erythema	
Discriminatory signs	The sharp demarcation of plaques, with clinically normal uninvolved skin in between (as occurs in psoriasis at other body sites). The scale produced has the appearance of silvery flakes.	Greasier yellowish-brown scale or crusting, and lesions that are usually more diffuse than in psoriasis
Associated features	Psoriasis at other sites, especially elbows, knees, and sacrum. However, scalp involvement may be an isolated feature.	Seborrhoeic dermatitis at other sites, especially mid-facial, eyebrows, and central chest. Associated otitis externa is more common in seborrhoeic dermatitis but can occur in psoriasis and is not diagnostic.
Important tests	None	Scalp scale may have profuse yeast spores and hyphae (*Pityrosporum ovale*) visualized on microscopy.
Treatment differences	Dithranol (anthralin), vitamin D analogues	Topical anti-yeast imidazole shampoos or creams

Further reading:
p. 6, p. 8, p. 26, p. 28, p. 40, p. 58, p. 60, pp. 80–84, p. 102, p. 110, p. 118, p. 120, p. 124, p. 174, p. 176.

References
Hersle K, Lindholm A, Mobaeken H, *et al.* Relationship of pityriasis amiantacea to psoriasis. *Dermatologica* 1979; **159**:245–50.
Knight AG. Pityriasis amiantacea: a clinical and histopathological investigation. *Clin Exp Dermatol* 1977; **2**:137–44.

Shuster S. The aetiology of dandruff and mode of action of therapeutic agents. *Br J Dermatol* 1984; **111**:235–42.

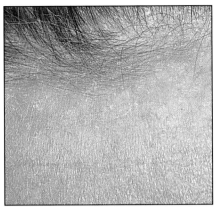

Figure 1.1 *Seborrhoeic dermatitis of the scalp margin: this shows the typical fine 'dandruff' pattern of scaling.*

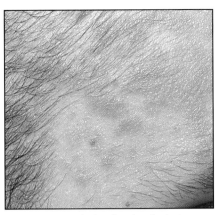

Figure 1.2 *Psoriasis of scalp: the lesions are typically discrete and more sharply defined than in seborrhoeic dermatitis.*

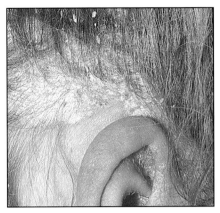

Figure 1.3 *Psoriasis of scalp: this demonstrates the silvery colour of scale, and underlying erythema (compare with Fig. 1.1).*

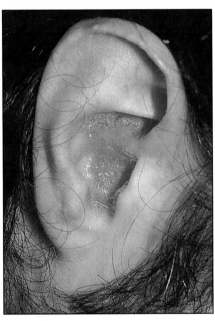

Figure 1.4 *Psoriasis of external auditory canal. This is a common site for either of these disorders. In this case, the degree of erythema and associated discrete scalp lesions favoured a diagnosis of psoriasis.*

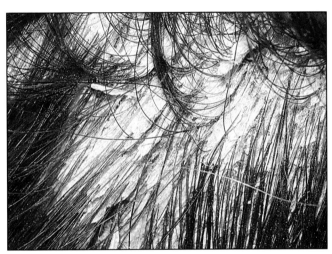

Figure 1.5 *Pityriasis amiantacea: thick 'asbestos-like' scaling can be a feature of several inflammatory dermatoses of scalp, most commonly of psoriasis.*

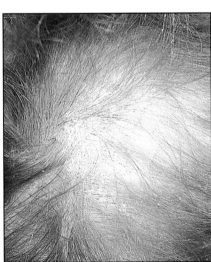

Figure 1.6 *Hair casts: these are visible as white specks in the hair.*

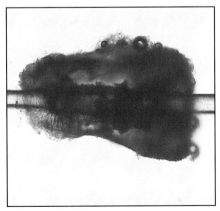

Figure 1.7 *Hair cast: this close-up view demonstrates the keratin bundle around the hair. The ability to slide a hair cast along the hair distinguishes it from the eggs (nits) of head lice.*

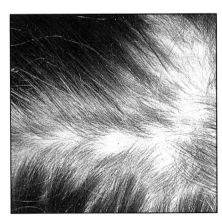

Figure 1.8 *Pityriasis amiantacea: some degree of permanent scarring may occur in up to 90% of patients, who may wrongly blame this on the treatment used to remove scaling (see also p. 6).*

Common presenting feature: alopecia, the follicles remaining intact. Confusion is particularly likely when only the scalp margin is involved.

Rationale for comparison: an incorrect diagnosis will lead to inappropriate treatment, advice, and prognosis.

Other differential diagnoses: trichotillomania; triangular alopecia; male pattern baldness.

Conclusion and key points: traction alopecia is related to hair style and usually affects the frontal or temporal scalp margin alone. Causes include hair braiding, long plaits, and use of tight hair-rollers, etc. The patient describes gradual progressive hair thinning, rather than increased hair fall. Alopecia areata usually affects other sites on the scalp, and displays pathognomonic, exclamation-mark hairs in the active phase of hair loss.

Comparative features		
Disorder	**Alopecia areata**	**Traction alopecia**
Age	Any	Any where mechanical hair styling is used
Sex	Either	Mainly female but some cultural hair styling methods may affect males also
Family history	May be positive for alopecia areata or other autoimmune disease	Non-specific
Sites	Any part of scalp; potential confusion is most likely to occur with the marginal pattern (ophiasis)	Mostly marginal, especially above ears and frontal areas
Symptoms	Usually none. The disorder may be discovered by a hairdresser rather than by the patient. Occasionally, itch is a feature at the onset. In alopecia areata of rapid onset and progression, patients will report increased hair fall and reduced hair density.	None. The history is of progressive thinning of hair rather than hair falling out excessively, and there are no other symptoms.
Signs common to both	Alopecia with intact (non-scarred) follicles	
Discriminatory signs	Typically disc-shaped areas of hair loss with smooth scalp or fine vellus hairs. Exclamation mark hairs are pathognomonic. 'Cadaverized' hairs (see Fig. 3.1) and easily kinked hairs may be present. Selective sparing of white hairs, or white regrowth, are both common.	The diagnosis is usually apparent from the hair style, and the lack of lesions at other parts of the scalp. Hairs are sparse but most are of normal length; some short damaged hairs may be apparent.
Associated features	Alopecia areata at other sites (beard area, eyebrows, eyelashes, body, limbs), sometimes nail pitting	In some patients with braided hair, there may be other cultural hair care damage (e.g. folliculitis due to hot oil).
Important tests	None, possibly thyroid function if clinically indicated	None

Further reading

pp. 6–10.

References

Anderson I. Alopecia areata. A clinical study. *BMJ* 1950; **ii**:250–4.

Fielder VC. Treatment of alopecia areata. *Dermatol Clinics* 1996; **14**:733–8.

Hoffmann R, Happle R. Topical immunotherapy in alopecia areata. *Dermatol Clinics* 1996; **14**:739–44.

Miller JA, Winkelmann RK. Alopecia areata. *Arch Dermatol* 1963; **88**:290–7.

Rook AJ. Common baldness and alopecia areata. *Recent Adv Dermatol* 1977; **4**:223–44.

Trachimas C, Sperling LC, Skelton HG, *et al.* Clinical and histologic findings in temporal triangular alopecia. *J Am Acad Dermatol* 1994; **31**:205–9.

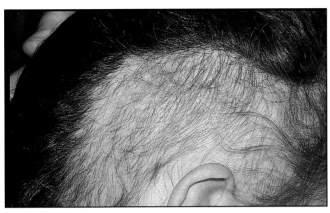

Figure 2.1 *Alopecia areata, showing the ophiasis pattern of marginal alopecia. Traction alopecia is also often marginal, but less sharply defined and does not extend as far into the scalp. Marginal alopecia in the occipital distribution is a typical site for alopecia areata, but either disorder may affect the temporal region.*

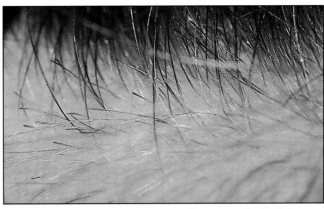

Figure 2.2 *Alopecia areata, showing a discrete patch of hair loss with pathognomonic exclamation-mark hairs.*

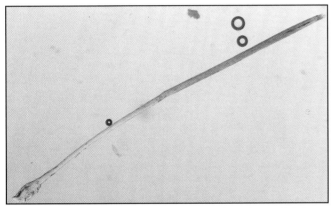

Figure 2.3 *Alopecia areata: microscopy of exclamation-mark hair showing fine, pale, dystrophic, basal hair shaft.*

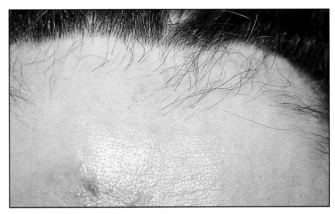

Figure 2.4 *Traction alopecia at the anterior scalp margin, demonstrating sparse hairs and a narrow zone of alopecia (compare with Fig. 2.1).*

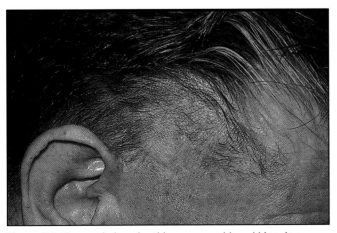

Figure 2.5 *Temporal alopecia: this was caused by rubbing, in a patient with atopic dermatitis. Note the underlying erythema and lichenification, neither of which are features of alopecia areata or simple traction alopecia.*

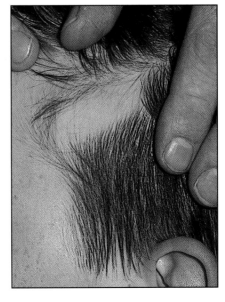

Figure 2.6
Triangular alopecia. This disorder, which is permanent but remains localized to the temples, is usually apparent in childhood, and may be misdiagnosed as alopecia areata. Residual fine vellus hairs are usually present.

3 Alopecia areata v. scarring alopecias

Common presenting feature: localized patches of alopecia.

Rationale for comparison: this is a comparison of a specific disorder versus a physical sign which may occur in several dermatoses. It is a frequent diagnostic problem and potentially of great significance, as scarring alopecia may be a feature of systemic diseases such as lupus erythematosus. Scarring alopecias all have the common sign of follicular scarring, which indicates irreversible hair loss. This is therefore an indication for aggressive therapy to prevent further scarring.

Other differential diagnoses: common causes of scarring alopecia are listed in the Table. The progressive inflammatory types are the most likely to be confused with alopecia areata, and may also be confused with tinea capitis, psoriasis, and seborrhoeic dermatitis (all of which may rarely lead to focal scarring in some individuals).

Conclusion and key points: follicular scarring is a readily recognized physical sign, which is often preceded or accompanied by evidence of active inflammation, such as erythema or pustule formation. The intact follicular openings of non-scarring disorders, such as alopecia areata, are easily differentiated, although the site of the follicular pores does decrease in long-standing alopecia areata. Distinguishing between the various causes of scarring alopecia is not always easy on the appearance alone, though some causes (e.g. nuchal acne keloid) are clinically characteristic. Biopsy and immunofluorescence of an active lesion is usually required to distinguish between the various inflammatory and immunobullous causes, and occasionally to exclude or classify neoplastic causes. A firm diagnosis is important for prognostic reasons.

Comparative features		
Disorder	**Alopecia areata**	**Scarring alopecia (inflammatory types with prominent scarring)**
Age	Any	Adult
Sex	Either	Either
Family history	May be positive for alopecia areata, thyroid disease, or other organ-specific autoimmune disorders	May be positive in lupus erythematosus, in which case consider inherited complement deficiency
Sites	Any. Some patterns strongly suggest this diagnosis e.g. marginal alopecia (ophiasis).	Any. Most types are not usually marginal (with the exception of nuchal acne keloid).
Symptoms	None/mild itch at onset	Some causes produce significant itch or tenderness.
Signs common to both	Localised patches of alopecia	
Discriminatory signs	Follicles are intact. Typical features (which may not all be present) include: exclamation mark hairs, selective sparing of white hairs, 'cadaverized' hairs, and easily kinked hairs. There may be mild localized scalp erythema at onset, or at the margin of an expanding patch of alopecia.	Active follicular inflammation may be present in affected areas or elsewhere on the scalp, e.g, follicular erythema (especially lupus erythematosus, lichen planus), follicular pustules (especially folliculitis decalvans), follicular crusting.
Associated features	May be involvement of other sites e.g. eyebrows, beard, nails (fine pitting). Concurrent thyroid disease is occasionally demonstrated.	Depends on cause (see Table). Always consider lupus erythematosus and lichen planus, and look for supportive evidence (rash at other sites, nailfold changes in lupus erythematosus, mucosal lesions in lichen planus).
Important tests	Usually none; thyroid function tests if clinically indicated	Exclude pyogenic and fungal infections (especially cattle ringworm) by swabs from pustules and mycology of affected hairs. For adult onset scarring alopecia, serology (antinuclear antibody etc., complement levels) and scalp biopsy including direct immunofluorescence are indicated unless there is a clear history of an obvious cause (e.g. trauma, burn).

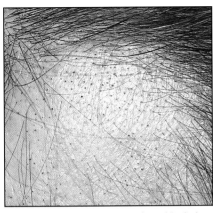

Figure 3.1 *Alopecia areata: these black dots are damaged ('cadaverized') hairs, and clearly demonstrate that the follicles are still present.*

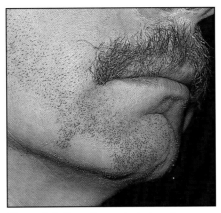

Figure 3.2 *Alopecia areata in beard area: there is hair loss without scarring.*

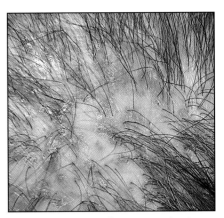

Figure 3.3 *Lupus erythematosus, showing loss of follicles, perifollicular erythema, and keratosis. Lichen planus of scalp is very similar.*

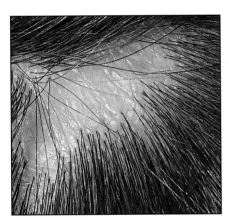

Figure 3.4 *Pseudopelade, showing circumscribed areas of scarring alopecia.*

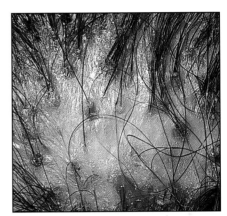

Figure 3.5 *Folliculitis decalvans, showing scarring, pustules, and clumping of hairs.*

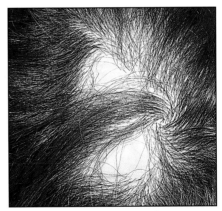

Figure 3.6 *Aplasia cutis: circumscribed scarring present in infancy, and persisting in adult life.*

Causes of scarring alopecia	
Inflammatory and idiopathic dermatoses	Discoid lupus erythematosus*, lichen planus*, dermatomyositis, scleroderma*, pseudopelade*, folliculitis decalvans*, nuchal acne keloid
Bullous disorders	Cicatricial pemphigoid, porphyria cutanea tarda, epidermolysis bullosa
Infections	Bacterial folliculitis*, tinea**, herpes zoster
External injury	Burns, wounds, radiotherapy
Neoplastic	Skin tumours and metastases to the skin
Developmental disorders	Naevus sebaceous (p. 12), aplasia cutis

*Most likely to be confused with alopecia areata
**Tinea due to *T. tonsurans* is most likely to be confused with alopecia areata, but kerion due to *T. verrucosum* (cattle ringworm) is most likely to scar

Further reading:
p. 4, p. 8, p. 10, p. 30.

References
Headington JT. Cicatricial alopecia. *Dermatol Clinics* 1996; **14**:773–82.
Newton RC, *et al.* Scarring alopecia. *Dermatol Clinics* 1987; **5**:603–18.
Werth VP. Incidence of alopecia areata in lupus erythematosus. *Arch Dermatol* 1992; **128**:368–71.
Wilson CL, *et al.* Scarring alopecia in discoid lupus erythematosus. *Br J Dermatol* 1992; **126**:307–14.

Common presenting feature: patches of alopecia with broken hairs.

Rationale for comparison: it is important to identify tinea capitis, as it is potentially infectious, readily treatable, and can cause permanent alopecia.

Other differential diagnoses: trichotillomania; hair loss following inflammatory dermatoses (e.g. psoriasis, pityriasis amiantacea).

Conclusion and key points: typical cat and dog ringworm in humans is easily differentiated from alopecia areata by the presence of greyish fine scaling and matted, broken-off hairs. These types fluoresce under Wood's light but other types do not; a negative Wood's light examination therefore does not exclude scalp tinea. 'Black dot' tinea (*Trichophyton tonsurans*) is less easy to distinguish, as hairs break below the skin surface and may look like the cadaverised hairs of alopecia areata. This type of scalp ringworm is more common in Afro-Caribbean children. Cattle ringworm causes a much more inflammatory disorder which is confused with pyogenic infection rather than with alopecia areata, and which may cause scarring alopecia (Fig. 4.6 and see also p. 6).

Comparative features		
Disorder	**Alopecia areata in children**	**Tinea capitis in children**
Age	Any (also occurs in adults)	Any. Scalp ringworm acquired from cats or dogs is much more common in children than in adults, but cattle ringworm is more frequent in adults than in children.
Sex	Either	
Family history	May be positive but usually historical	Often affects siblings concurrently, either due to person-to-person spread, or more commonly due to the same animal source
Sites	Any part of scalp	
Symptoms	None, occasionally mild itch. Rapid hair fall noted in conjunction with alopecia	None, itch
Signs common to both	Patch(es) of alopecia	
Discriminatory signs	Most hairs in the affected skin are totally lost, but some are broken off. Residual fine downy hair may remain in older lesions. Exclamation-mark hairs (Fig. 2.2) are pathognomonic; the scalp skin is normal.	Typical cat and dog tinea capitis leaves broken hairs. The lower part of the hair shaft is intact and coated with fungus, hence has a greyish matted appearance. The 'black dot' type, usually caused by *T. tonsurans*, is less common and more easily confused with alopecia areata. Scalp ringworm caused by *T. verrucosum* (usually from cattle) produces a pustular and inflammatory reaction and is less likely to be confused with alopecia areata.
Associated features	May be alopecia of eyebrows, eyelashes; occasionally nail pitting	May be classic ringworm lesions elsewhere. Typically the family pet is also affected.
Important tests	None	Examination under Wood's light; cat or dog ringworm fluoresces but other forms of ringworm do not, hence a negative result does not exclude tinea. Mycological examination of affected hair shafts is required.

Further reading:
p. 4, p. 6, p. 10, p. 68, p. 96, p. 120, p. 170, p. 172.

References
Fuller LC, Child FC, Higgins EM. Tinea capitis in south-east London: an outbreak of *Trichophyton tonsurans* infection. *Br J Dermatol* 1997; **136**:139.
Levy ML. Disorders of the hair and scalp in children. *Pediatr Clin N Am* 1991; **38**:905–19.

MacKenzie DWR. Hairbrush technique in detection and eradication of non-fluorescent scalp ringworm. *BMJ* 1963; **ii**:363–5.
Muller SA. Trichotillomania. *Dermatol Clinics* 1987; **5**:595–601.
Pipkin JL. Tinea capitis in adults and adolescence. *Arch Dermatol* 1952; **66**:9–40.
Sahn EE. Alopecia areata in childhood. *Semin Dermatol* 1995; **14**:9–14.

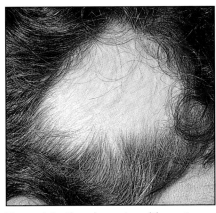

Figure 4.1 *Alopecia areata: with scanty regrowth of white hairs, a common feature.*

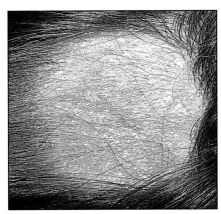

Figure 4.2 *Tinea capitis: showing a fairly well-demarcated area of broken-off hairs, coated with greyish-coloured masses of fungi.*

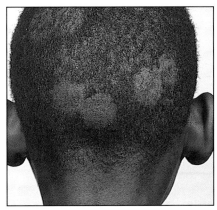

Figure 4.3 Trichophyton tonsurans *infection in a child: note the 'black dot' pattern in which hairs have broken at or below the scalp surface, and do not therefore demonstrate the coated appearance of the short broken hairs that occur in cat or dog ringworm (photograph kindly provided by Dr Elisabeth Higgins).*

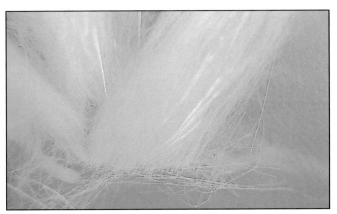

Figure 4.4 *Wood's light examination of hairs (in this case, white cat fur): this demonstrates fluorescence of* Trichophyton canis *on individual slightly thickened hairs.*

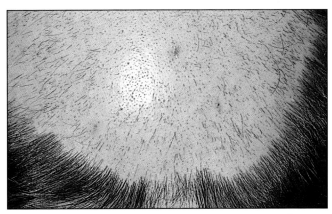

Figure 4.5 *Trichotillomania: note the stubbly broken hairs of variable length without the empty follicles of alopecia areata or the coated appearance of tinea capitis.*

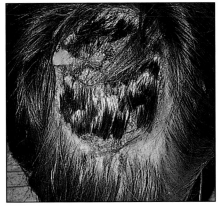

Figure 4.6 *Kerion (cattle ringworm) of scalp: this is a much more inflammatory disorder than tinea capitis due to cat or dog ringworm.*

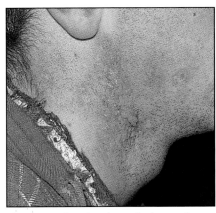

Figure 4.7 *Scarring due to kerion on the neck of a young man.*

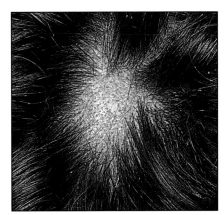

Figure 4.8 *Alopecia due to psoriasis. In this case the follicles are intact and regrowth occurred.*

Common presenting feature: increased hair fall and reduced hair density causing hair thinning without discrete patches of alopecia.

Rationale for comparison: these two disorders may be difficult to differentiate on examination but preceding events may provide the diagnosis. Their respective prognoses and treatments are different.

Other differential diagnoses: androgenetic alopecia; trichotillomania; metabolic alopecia (thyroid disease); anagen effluvium (chemotherapy); congenital hair disorders in younger patients (e.g. monilethrix).

Conclusion and key points: occasionally an episode of alopecia areata appears to follow a psychologically stressful event after an interval of a few weeks. A longer interval is not generally accepted as consistent with a causal relationship. In telogen effluvium, a wave of hair fall occurs following a specific trigger, such as pregnancy or illness. This occurs because hairs remain in the telogen (resting) phase of the follicular cycle during the pregnancy or illness, and thus a larger than normal number of hairs subsequently enter the catagen (hair loss) phase together, when the causative stimulus is no longer present. New growth is seen after a further 8 weeks. A chronic form of telogen effluvium in middle-aged women has also been described recently. No treatment is required or useful in telogen effluvium, other than strong reassurance that improvement will occur spontaneously.

Comparative features		
Disorder	**Diffuse alopecia areata**	**Telogen effluvium**
Age	Any	
Sex	Either	Either (common after pregnancy)
Family history	May be positive for alopecia areata, thyroid disease, or other autoimmune disease	Non-specific
Sites	Diffuse scalp involment; may affect other body sites (see below)	Diffuse scalp. Regrowth is often most apparent at the forehead margin.
Symptoms	Usually none except sudden onset of hair loss, which is usually progressive. Some patients report itch at the onset.	None, except sudden onset of hair loss, which stops after about 2 months
Signs common to both	Diffuse hair thinning with history of rapid hair fall, follicles intact	
Discriminatory signs	May be none as specific changes are often scanty. Exclamation-mark hairs (Fig. 2.2) or 'cadaverized' hairs may be visible. Small groups of empty follicles may be visible. Alopecia areata may selectively leave white hairs unaffected.	Discrete areas of total loss are not a feature.
Associated features	Usually none. Nail pits, or alopecia at other body sites (e.g. eyebrows, eyelashes, beard) may be present.	Identified from history; usually postpartum or following a severe infection or other illness, and associated with dramatic rate of hair loss
Important tests	Hair pluck demonstrates dystrophic telogen hairs during the phase of active loss. Thyroid function tests may be clinically indicated.	Hair pluck reveals increased proportion of morphologically normal telogen hairs (30–50%).

Further reading:
p. 4, p. 6, p. 8.

References
Brodin MB. Drug related alopecia. *Dermatol Clinics* 1987; **5**:571–9.
Kligman AM. Pathologic dynamics of human hair loss. I. Telogen effluvium. *Arch Dermatol* 1961; **83**:175–95.
Piacquadio DJ, *et al.* Obesity and female androgenic alopecia: a cause and an effect? *J Am Acad Dermatol* 1994; **30**:1028–30.

Schiff BL, Kern AB. Study of post-partum alopecia. *Arch Dermatol* 1963; **87**:609–11.
Whiting DA. Chronic telogen effluvium: increased scalp hair shedding in middle-aged women. *J Am Acad Dermatol* 1996; **35**:899–906.

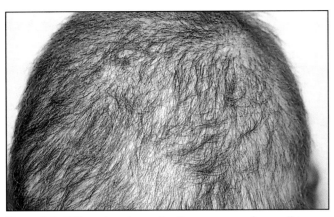

Causes of telogen effluvium	
Hormonal	Post-pregnancy, post-oral contraceptive
Drugs	Acute overdose, anticoagulants, cimetidine, anticonvulsants
Metabolic	Strict dieting, thyrotoxicosis
Other causes	Severe illness, injury, blood loss, fever

Figure 5.1 *Diffuse alopecia areata: the appearance from a distance is of non-specific hair thinning.*

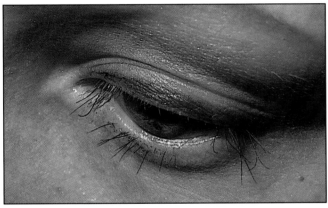

Figure 5.2 *Loss of hair from sites such as eyebrows or eyelashes, as shown here, may be a useful diagnostic pointer to alopecia areata when there is clinical doubt (but may also be plucked-out in trichotillomania).*

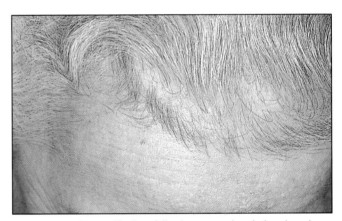

Figure 5.3 *Telogen effluvium following severe drug-induced erythema multiforme, which also caused significant forehead scarring. A synchronized cohort of regrowing hairs of equal lengths is most easily visible at the frontal hair margin.*

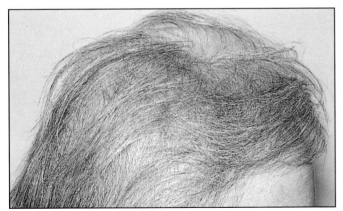

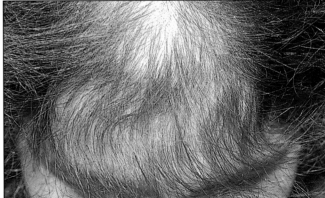

Figures 5.4 and 5.5 *Androgenetic alopecia may be similar in general appearance to diffuse alopecia areata or telogen effluvium, but there is no history of profuse hair fall, and the frontal margin is usually relatively spared.*

6 Melanocytic naevus ('mole') v. organoid naevus (naevus sebaceus)

Common presenting feature: soft to firm, cobblestoned or papillomatous, scalp nodules.

Rationale for comparison: these two disorders are commonly confused. Several types of neoplasm may arise in organoid naevi. Melanocytic naevi of scalp are benign but are frequently present in patients with numerous naevi at other sites.

Other differential diagnoses: viral warts (commonly confused with these diagnoses); skin appendage neoplasia; epidermal naevi; scalp metastases.

Conclusion and key points: scalp melanocytic naevi do not need to be removed unless they are symptomatic (e.g. they catch on hairbrushes). They may occur as part of the dysplastic naevus syndrome in which patients have multiple atypical naevi. Organoid naevi are hamartomas which can be differentiated by their orange colour, absence or marked paucity of hairs growing through the lesion, and tendency to become thicker at puberty. As they may be complicated by a variety of appendage neoplasms and occasionally basal cell carcinomas, prophylactic removal is sensible. Extensive organoid naevi may be associated with other congenital abnormalities.

Comparative features		
Disorder	**Scalp melanocytic naevus**	**Scalp organoid naevus (naevus sebaceus)**
Age	Usually not apparent until second decade	Present in infancy as an area of permanent alopecia, but sometimes first noticed at puberty when the surface becomes more cobblestoned or warty
Sex	Either	
Family history	May occur in familial dysplastic naevus syndrome	Non-specific
Sites	Any part of scalp	
Symptoms	None, unless traumatized	None unless traumatized. Persistent crusting of the surface suggests that a secondary neoplasm has developed within the organoid naevus.
Signs common to both	Cobblestoned/papillomatous nodule	
Discriminatory signs	Usually more dome shaped and softer than organoid naevi. Most less than 1 cm in diameter. Hairs are typically present but variable in amount. Pigment varies, but often there is only a fine dusting of brown pigment.	Orange colour. Typically this is a cobblestoned plaque, which may have spikier verrucous areas or more nodular areas often 2 cm or greater in diameter. Hairs are typically absent although some naevi contain a few intact hairs.
Associated features	Occasionally atypical naevi at other sites, or more naevi than expected for the age group	Usually none
Important tests	None routinely required. Shave biopsy may be necessary for lesions which catch on hairbrushes, and, rarely, formal excision if clinically atypical.	Best to excise at puberty/young adult age group; basal cell carcinoma may develop in up to 15% of cases

Further reading:
p. 46, p. 50, p. 160, p. 162.

References

Bataille V, *et al*. Risk of cutaneous melanoma in relation to the number, types and sites of naevi. A case control study. *Br J Cancer* 1996; **73**:1605–11.

Constant E, Davis DG. The premalignant nature of the nevus sebaceus of Jadassohn. *Plast Reconstr Surg* 1972; **50**:257–9.

Wilson–Jones E, Heyl T. Naevus sebaceus:a report of 140 cases with special regard to the development of secondary malignant tumours. *Br J Dermatol* 1970; **82**:99–117.

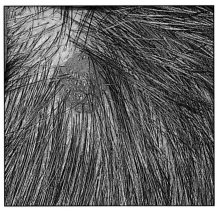

Figure 6.1 *Pigmented scalp naevus: this is similar to naevi at more typical body sites.*

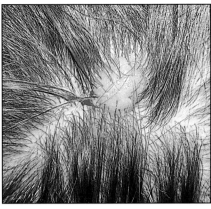

Figure 6.2 *Flesh-coloured scalp melanocytic naevus: lack of significant pigment is common in scalp naevi.*

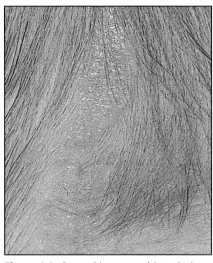

Figure 6.3 *Organoid naevus with typical orange colour and warty surface.*

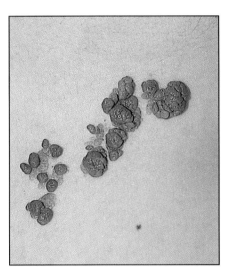

Figure 6.4 *Epidermal naevi on the neck (a more typical site than within the scalp): these may look similar to ordinary pigment naevi but are typically linear.*

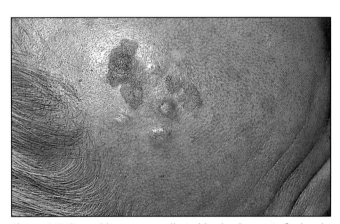

Figure 6.5 *Organoid naevus complicated by development of a basal cell carcinoma at the anterior pole.*

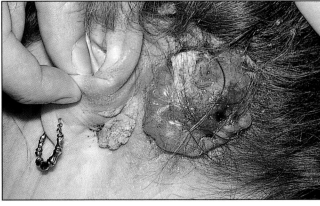

Figure 6.6 *Organoid naevus with a large basal cell carcinoma arising within it.*

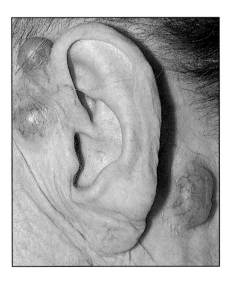

Figure 6.7 *Cylindroma: the scalp is also a frequent site for other skin appendage neoplasms, such as the cylindroma (turban tumour) shown here.*

13

7 Geographical tongue v. other causes of sore tongue

Common presenting feature: sore tongue.

Rationale for comparison: geographical tongue (migratory glossitis) is a clinically characteristic disorder which may occur in 1–2% of the population, though it is usually asymptomatic. A firm clinical diagnosis of geographical tongue excludes the need for systemic investigations and patients can be reassured about the benign nature of the condition.

Other differential diagnoses: candidosis; aphthous ulceration and rarer forms of recurrent ulceration; lichen planus; vitamin deficiencies; allergy to dental materials, and denture sore mouth; food allergies; drug reactions.

Conclusion and key points: the visible changes in geographical tongue vary from day to day. The characteristic lesions are discrete annular and arciform areas which are predominantly around the tip of the tongue but which may occur on the buccal mucosa or palate. Similar appearances may be seen in patients with generalized pustular psoriasis or Reiter's syndrome. The differential diagnosis includes candidal infection, which is most common in smokers, patients who wear dentures, and immunosuppressed individuals. Where there is diagnostic doubt, it is useful to treat empirically with a topical imidazole, as culture of organisms can be difficult in some candidal eruptions, such as median rhomboid glossitis. Extensive screening for deficiencies and allergies is unnecessary when the physical signs are characteristic.

Comparative features		
Disorder	**Geographical tongue**	**Other causes of sore tongue**
Age	Any, especially peak early adulthood	Any, especially middle-age onwards
Sex	Female predominance	
Family history	Occasionally present	Non-specific
Sites	Mainly anterior part of tongue	Mostly, diffuse or central tongue
Symptoms	Sore tongue, aggravated by acidic or spicy foods	
Signs common to both	May be no visible abnormality or non-specific erythema	
Discriminatory signs	Annular or arciform red or off-white lesions, typically variable from day to day. They may be atrophic in appearance.	Signs depend on the underlying disorder. Confluent and persistent erythema suggests *candida*, vitamin deficiency, or rarities such as necrolytic migratory erythema. An abnormally red area with papillary atrophy in the centre of the tongue suggests median rhomboid glossitis.
Associated features	None in most patients. Can occur in conjunction with severe, pustular psoriasis or Reiter's syndrome	Often none. May be overt candidosis of other sites in some patients, or other signs of malnutrition or vitamin deficiency
Important tests	None	Bacteriology samples for *Candida*. Full blood count and indices. Others as indicated from concomitant symptoms

Further reading:
p. 16, p. 18.

References
Budzt–Jorgensen E. Oral mucosal lesions associated with the wearing of removable dentures. *J Oral Pathol* 1981; **10**:65–80.
Halperin V, *et al.* The occurrence of Fordyce spots, benign migratory glossitis, median rhomboid glossitis, and fissured tongue in 2,478 dental patients. *Oral Surg* 1974; **37**:872.

Huang W, Rothe MJ, Grant–Kels JM. The burning mouth syndrome. *J Am Acad Dermatol* 1996; **34**:91–8.
Marks R, Radden BG. Geographic tongue: a clinico-pathological review. *Aust J Dermatol* 1981; **22**:75–9.
Van der Waal N. Candida albicans in median rhomboid glossitis: a post mortem study. *Int J Oral Maxillofacial Surg* 1986; **15**:322–5.

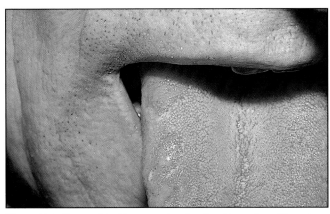

Figure 7.1 *Geographical tongue, showing focal loss of papillae at the border of the tongue.*

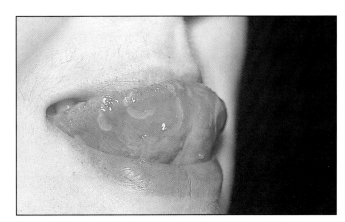

Figure 7.2 *Geographical tongue: an arciform pattern as shown here is diagnostic.*

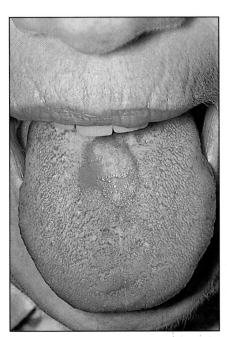

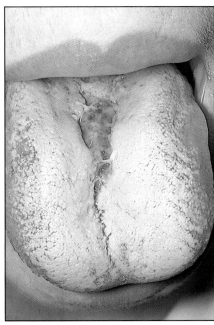

Figures 7.3 and 7.4 *Median rhomboid glossitis, a manifestation of candidosis.*

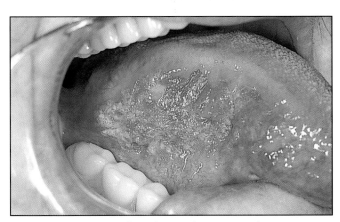

Figure 7.5 *Squamous cell carcinoma of tongue may be asymptomatic but is palpably indurated (photograph kindly provided by Mr G. Putnam).*

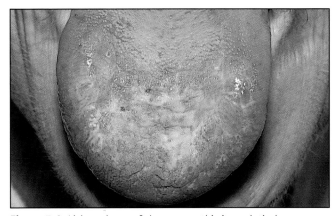

Figure 7.6 *Lichen planus of the tongue: this is a relatively uncommon site, but the streaky white lesions are typical (see also p. 16).*

8 Lichen planus and lichenoid plaques v. leukoplakia

Common presenting feature: white lines or patches of oral mucosa.

Rationale for comparison: these conditions share several physical signs but differ in the investigations required, treatment, and outcome.

Other differential diagnoses: bite line; mechanical damage from rough fillings; geographical tongue (migratory glossitis, see p. 14); candidal infection; oral hairy leukoplakia (a feature of AIDS).

Conclusion and key points: lichen planus (LP) of the buccal mucosa is usually a symmetrical and often asymptomatic disorder which may occur in isolation, but it is also present in about 75% of patients with cutaneous lichen planus. Lichenoid reactions are a relatively non-specific response to various forms of injury to the buccal mucosa; causes include reactions to dental amalgam, in which case the lesions affect buccal mucosa or the side of the tongue in proximity to filled teeth. Leukoplakia is an asymmetrical disorder, which is premalignant; it should always be excluded by biopsy if the floor of the mouth is involved.

Comparative features		
Disorder	**Lichen planus (LP) and lichenoid reactions**	**Leukoplakia**
Age	Adult	
Sex	Either	
Family history	Rarely positive for cutaneous lichen planus	Negative
Sites	Usually buccal. When associated with cutaneous LP, the lips and tongue may be affected. Lichenoid reactions due to mercury in amalgams may affect the buccal mucosa and tongue adjacent to an old amalgam dental filling, but do not generally occur adjacent to all fillings.	Any. Floor of mouth and palatal involvement in isolation are more typical of leukoplakia than of LP.
Symptoms	Occasionally none; usually painful	Usually none; may be painful
Signs common to both	White striae, patches of oral mucosa	
Discriminatory signs	Typically a lace-like reticulate pattern is present, which is usually more delicate in oral LP compared with lichenoid reactions. Erosions may be present. Oral LP in patients with cutaneous LP is usually symmetrical, but lichenoid amalgam reactions are asymmetrical.	Usually an asymmetrical, confluent, mixed white and red plaque. The affected mucosa has a more lobular pattern and less well defined reticulate striae than in LP. There may be an erythematous component or a raised cobblestoned surface.
Associated features	May be cutaneous lichen planus	Frequently associated with cigarette-smoking
Important tests	Patch test to ammoniated mercury if LP is localized adjacent to an amalgam filling and is not associated with cutaneous LP. Biopsy if LP is chronic or if new features develop, especially if there is sustained erosion, as secondary development of squamous cell carcinoma can occur.	Biopsy

Further reading:
p. 81 (Fig. 40.4), p. 150.

References
Bouquot JE. Reviewing oral leukoplakia: clinical concepts for the 1990s. *J Am Dental Assoc* 1991; **122**:80–2.
Bouquot JE. Oral leukoplakia and erythroleukoplakia: a review and update. *Pract Periodontics Aesthet Dent* 1994; **6**:9–17.
Husak R, Garbe C, Orfanos CE. Oral hairy leukoplakia in 71 HIV-seropositive patients: clinical symptoms, relationship to immunologic status, and prognostic significance. *J Am Acad Dermatol* 1996; **35**:928–34.

Ibbotson SH, Speight EL, McLeod RI, Smart ER, Lawrence CM. The relevance and effect of amalgam replacement in subjects with oral lichenoid reactions. *Br J Dermatol* 1996; **134**:420–3.
Resnick L, Herbst JS, Raab–Traub N. Oral hairy leukoplakia. *J Am Acad Dermatol* 1990; **22**:1278–82.
Scully C, Elkom M. Lichen planus. Review and update on pathogenesis. *J Oral Pathol* 1985; **14**:431–58.

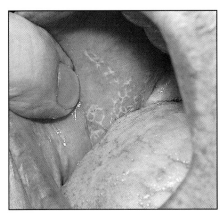

Figure 8.1 *Oral lichen planus: this shows the typical lace-like reticulate pattern.*

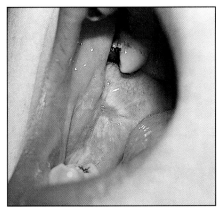

Figure 8.2 *Oral lichenoid reaction due to mercury in dental amalgam: this has a less delicate appearance and is in obvious approximation to a dental filling.*

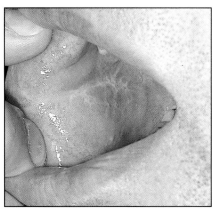

Figure 8.3 *Linear lichenoid appearance, due to repeated trauma of teeth clenching ('bite line').*

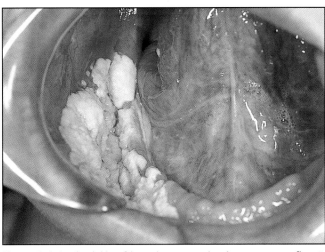

Figure 8.4 *Leukoplakia of buccal mucosa, showing a more confluent white area with lobulated margin.*

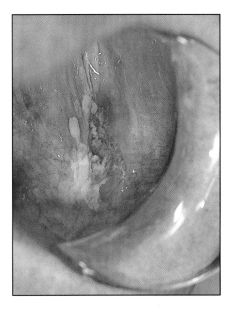

Figure 8.5 *Leukoplakia due to carcinoma in situ and early invasive carcinoma.*

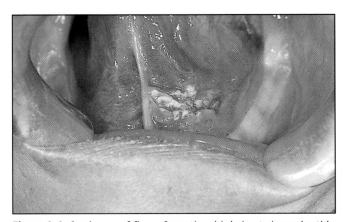

Figure 8.6 *Carcinoma of floor of mouth, with indurated margin: this is an unlikely site for lichen planus (Figs. 8.4, 8.5 and 8.6 kindly provided by Mr G. Putnam).*

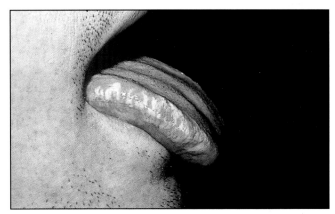

Figure 8.7 *Oral hairy leukoplakia: a sign of AIDS. Concomitant Kaposi's sarcoma of the palate was present.*

9 Fordyce spots v. *Candida* infection

Common presenting feature: punctate whitish lesions of oral mucosa or lips.

Rationale for comparison: Fordyce spots are a normal variant, for which no treatment is required.

Other differential diagnoses: lichen planus.

Conclusion and key points: Fordyce spots are a common normal variant which can be recognized by their typical site distribution, yellowish colour, static nature, and lack of symptoms.

Comparative features		
Disorder	**Fordyce spots**	**Candidosis**
Age	Teens onwards	Any
Sex	Either	
Family history	Non-specific	
Sites	Inside vermilion border, especially lateral aspects of upper lip, and buccal mucosa	Palatal, buccal, tongue, and gingival mucosa
Symptoms	None	Usually burning; may be none or just dryness
Signs common to both	Papular lesions of oral mucosa	
Discriminatory signs	Yellowish colour, small size and monomorphic, no erythematous component, fixed position	White colour, coalescing lesions, erythematous background, can be scraped off
Associated features	Occasionally occur at extraoral sites (especially genital)	There may be a history of antibiotic or corticosteroid (inhaled or oral) usage, diabetes, recent illness, or immunosuppression. Dentures, and any cause of dry mouth (drug-induced, sicca syndrome, local radiotherapy) also predispose to candidal infection. There may be associated perineal candidosis in babies and the elderly, vulval candidosis in women, or angular cheilitis.
Important tests	None	Culture to confirm diagnosis; investigate underlying causes.

Further reading:
p. 14, p. 16.

References
Dilley DC, Siegel MA, Budnick S. Diagnosing and treating common oral pathogens. *Ped Clin N Am* 1991; **38**:1227–64.
Greenspan D, Greenspan DS. Oral manifestations of HIV infection. *Dermatol Clinics* 1991; **9**:517–22.
Korting HC. Clinical spectrum of oral candidosis and its role in HIV-infected patients. *Mycoses* 1989; **32**(Suppl 2):23–9.

Miles AEW. Sebaceous glands in oral and lip mucosa. In: Montagna W, Ellis RA, Silver AF. *Advances in Biology of Skin*, Vol 4. *The sebaceous glands.* New York, Macmillan Company 1963:46–77.
Odds FC. *Candida* infections: an overview. *CRC Crit Rev Microbiol* 1987; **15**:1–5.

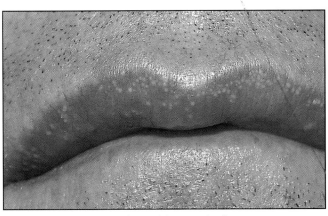

Figure 9.1 *Fordyce spots, located here on the lips.*

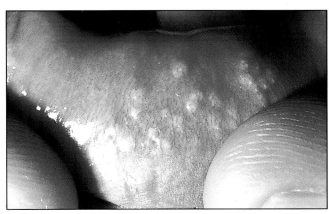

Figure 9.2 *Fordyce spots: close-up demonstrates uniform size and yellowish colour.*

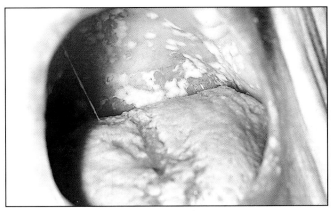

Figure 9.3 *Oral candidosis: there are irregular white plaques on the palate and median rhomboid glossitis of the tongue.*

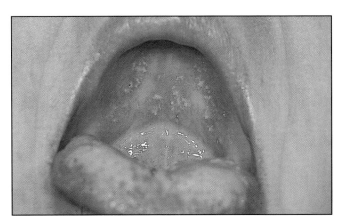

Figure 9.4 *Oral candidosis (same patient as in Fig. 7.4); it is common for lesions to be confined to the area under a denture as in this case.*

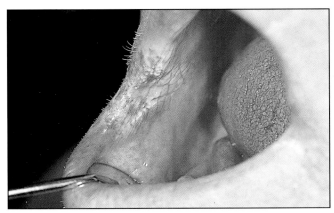

Figure 9.5 *Candidosis inside the commissure may mimic leukoplakia (p. 16, see also Fig 8.4) or lichen planus/lichenoid eruptions (photograph kindly provided by Mr G. Putnam).*

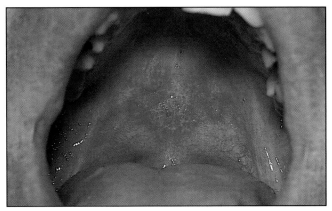

Figure 9.6 *Lichen planus of palate: the reticulate pattern and localized erythema differentiates this from candidal infection.*

10 Lips: Eczema v. actinic cheilitis

Common presenting feature: scaling and crusting of the lower lip.

Rationale for comparison: actinic cheilitis is frequently erroneously diagnosed and treated as eczema.

Other differential diagnoses: angular cheilitis; vanishing vermilion border; lupus erythematosus.

Conclusion and key points: scaling of the lower lip in middle-aged or elderly patients, which does not extend beyond the vermilion border, is usually due to actinic damage rather than eczema. Actinic keratoses may be present elsewhere but their detection is not required for the diagnosis. Angular cheilitis occurs at the corners of the mouth and is usually of mechanical origin, complicated by low-grade candidal infection, rather than being caused by dietary deficiencies which are often incorrectly blamed for the condition. Vanishing vermilion border (see Fig. 10.7 and the reference Mohareb *et al.* given below) is an asymptomatic condition of pale skin areas developing at the periphery of the vermilion of the lip.

Comparative features		
Disorder	**Actinic cheilitis**	**Lip eczema**
Age	Middle-age, elderly	Any
Sex	Mainly male	Either
Family history	Negative	
Sites	Lower lip. May be localized or affect the whole length of the lip, but the intraoral portion of the vermilion is spared	Mainly affects the lower lip unless an allergen is applied directly to the upper lip (e.g. in lipstick, lip salve)
Symptoms	Irritation, itch	
Signs common to both	Scaling, crusting of lower lip	
Discriminatory signs	Confined to the vermilion of the lip. The surface change is hyperkeratosis, erosion, or crusting rather than finer eczematous scaling. Skin thinning, due to sun-induced dermal atrophy, is also clinically apparent.	Spreads beyond the vermilion border onto adjacent skin even if due to lipstick etc. Clinical signs may be most prominent at the angles of mouth, especially if toothpastes are the cause. Oedema may be present during acute episodes.
Associated features	May be actinic keratoses at other exposed sites	None specifically
Important tests	Biopsy if thickened or persistent localized areas, as actinic cheilitis may be a precursor of squamous cell carcinoma of the lip.	Consider patch testing to investigate possible allergy to foods, cosmetics, topical medicaments, and toothpaste flavourings.

Further reading:
p. 14, p. 22, p. 24, p. 32, p. 38, p. 54, p. 76, p. 78, p. 154.

References
Daley TD, Gupta AK. Exfoliative cheilitis. *J Oral Path Oral Med* 1995; 24:177–9.
Mohareb R, Elkomy M, Hanna N. Study of a new anomaly of the vermilion border of the lip. *Br J Dermatol* 1975; **92**:559–61.

Scheman A. Contact allergy testing alternatives 1996. *Cutis* 1996; **57**:235–40.

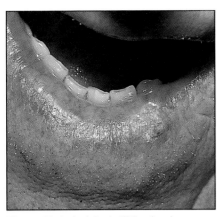

Figure 10.1 *Actinic cheilitis, showing crusting and colour variation of the lip with a focal area of discrete hyperkeratosis.*

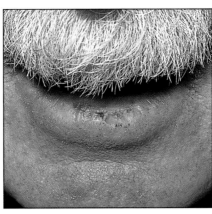

Figure 10.2 *Actinic cheilitis, showing erosion and adjacent crusting and atrophy.*

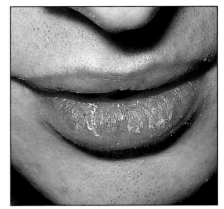

Figure 10.3 *Lip eczema, probably with some degree of abrading of the affected area with the upper incisors (lip chewing).*

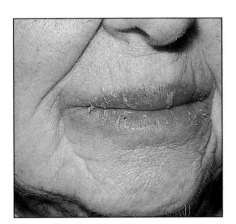

Figure 10.4 *Lip eczema due to a contact dermatitis to lip salve. Note the spread beyond the area of the vermilion border.*

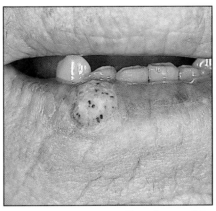

Figure 10.5 *Squamous cell carcinoma of lip and mild adjacent actinic cheilitis (photograph kindly provided by Mr G. Putnam).*

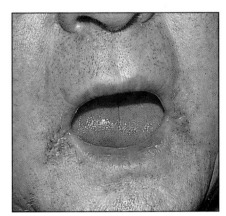

Figure 10.6 *Angular cheilitis due to poorly fitting dentures and secondary candidal infection.*

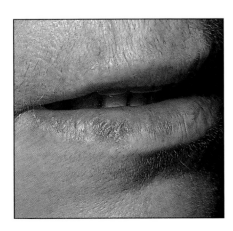

Figure 10.7 *Vanishing vermilion border. This disorder is probably not uncommon, with the appearance of focal marginal loss of colour from the lip. The disorder has no pathological significance.*

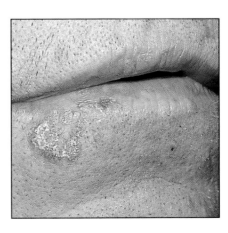

Figure 10.8 *Lupus erythematosus of lips: this is a discrete scaly lesion affecting the vermilion and adjacent skin. Note the atrophic scarring.*

II Lips: Lip-lick v. allergic contact eczema

Common presenting feature: eczema of lips.

Rationale for comparison: it is important to consider specific external causative factors as these may be avoidable.

Other differential diagnoses: median lip fissure; angular cheilitis; perioral dermatitis; contact urticaria.

Conclusion and key points: lip-lick eczema is an irritant dermatitis caused by contact with saliva. It can usually be differentiated from allergic dermatitis by distribution and morphology. Lip-lick eczema chiefly affects the circumoral skin more than the lips, and is typically sharply defined. However, the situation may be more complicated; a contact dermatitis may be aggravated by lip-licking, while some contact dermatitis is due to medicaments used to treat a lip-lick dermatitis.

Comparative features		
Disorder	**Lip-lick eczema**	**Allergic contact dermatitis of lips**
Age	Usually child	Any, mostly adult
Sex	Either	Either, but some causes are commoner in women (lip cosmetics)
Family history	May be atopic	Negative
Sites	Perioral, upper and lower lip	Vermilion and adjacent skin; upper and lower lips if due to lip salve, lipstick etc. Lower lip and angular area if due to toothpastes
Symptoms	Chronic itch and soreness with fissuring around lips	Itch, with erythema or swelling; may be intermittent or chronic
Signs common to both	Eczematous eruption of lips (erythema, scaling, fissures)	
Discriminatory signs	Distribution, sharp margin within limit of reach of the tongue. It is useful to observe the patient for lip licking during the consultation. The vermilion of the lip is relatively less affected.	Usually less well demarcated if chronic
Associated features	Affected children may be atopic. Parents are often not aware that the child licks lips. In young children the eruption may be asymmetrical due to dribbling or thumb sucking and may be associated with chronic paronychia of the thumb.	There may be a history of cosmetic reactions at other body sites, because flavourings in toothpastes, chewing gum, and sweets contain chemicals similar to those of certain cosmetic fragrance materials.
Important tests	May require patch tests	Patch test to appropriate allergens, e.g. lip salves, lipsticks, rubber, medicaments, constituents of creams, etc.

Further reading:
p. 20, p. 24, p. 32, p. 38, p. 76.

References
Fisher AA. *Contact dermatitis*, 3rd edn. Philadelphia, Lea and Febinger, 1986:791–5.

Hisa T, *et al.* Senile lip licking. *Dermatology* 1995; **191**:339–40.
Ophaswongse S, Maibach HI. Allergic contact cheilitis. *Contact dermatitis* 1995; **33**:365–70.

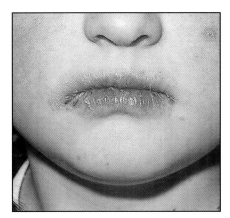

Figure 11.1 *Lip-lick eczema, showing typical age-group, distribution and sharp demarcation. This patient also had a positive patch test to cobalt, which is a common metal in household items.*

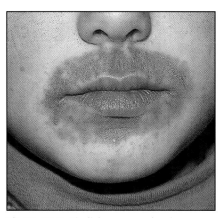

Figure 11.2 *Lip-lick eczema, showing unusually wide distribution but sharp demarcation, as in Fig. 11.1.*

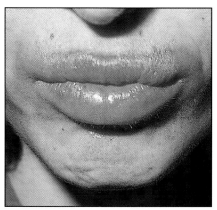

Figure 11.3 *Acute contact allergy to lipsalve: distribution is dictated by sites of application but usually produces a less sharply demarcated area of eczema compared with simple lip-lick allergy, probably due to the spread of the allergen onto the skin.*

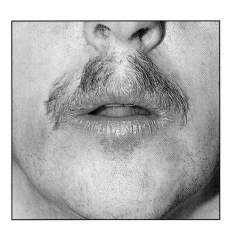

Figure 11.4 *Contact allergy to toothpaste, with typical involvement primarily of the angles of the mouth and lower lip.*

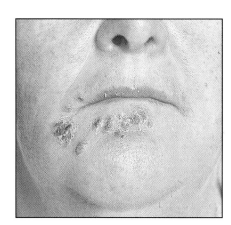

Figure 11.5 *Contact allergy to thiuram, a chemical used in rubber manufacture. The source was a dentist's rubber glove, which has caused a poorly demarcated area of reaction due to several points of contact.*

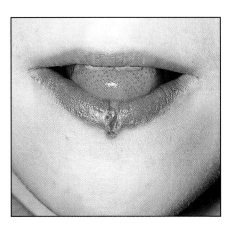

Figure 11.6 *Median lip fissure: this is a common problem, seen mainly in children.*

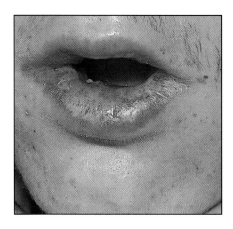

Figure 11.7 *Erythema multiforme affecting the lips alone: this may be confused with eczema or angioedema in the absence of typical cutaneous 'target' lesions.*

12 Lips: Angioedema v. contact urticaria

Common presenting feature: intermittent swelling of the lip(s).

Rationale for comparison: these two disorders may have different causes but result in a similar appearance. Contact urticaria may be prevented by identification and avoidance of a contact allergen. Angioedema is potentially life-threatening, particularly the hereditary form.

Other differential diagnoses: orofacial granulomatosis; Crohn's disease.

Conclusion and key points: angioedema is most striking when it occurs on lips or eyelids, but may also affect other body sites such as distal limbs. It occurs as part of a systemic urticarial process, usually with no specific identifiable trigger. In angioedema, extravasated tissue fluid is deeper and more intense than in urticaria and therefore causes deeper and longer-lasting swelling compared with the transient superficial erythema and weals of urticaria. Swelling which is transient and consistently confined to the lips may in fact be contact urticaria; this is most commonly caused by foods or, occasionally, by other items which are only in contact with lips. Causative allergens can generally be diagnosed by a careful clinical history.

More fixed swelling is usually due to orofacial granulomatosis or to Crohn's disease; the latter also causes intraoral changes. Repeated regular contact with an allergen may also produce chronic lip swelling, especially if there is secondary infection leading to lymphatic damage. Some foods, particularly protein allergens such as shellfish and peanuts, may cause localized lip swelling accompanied by other systemic symptoms such as wheeze and hypotension due to histamine release.

Comparative features		
Disorder	**Angioedema**	**Contact urticaria**
Age	Any, hereditary type usually presents before 30 years of age	Any, often children
Sex	Either	
Family history	Occasionally positive (if due to deficiency of C1 esterase inhibitor). Not all patients have angioedema of skin; some suffer abdominal symptoms or sudden death.	Non-specific
Sites	Lips, eyelids, other sites (face, limbs)	Lips; may affect other sites of direct contact
Symptoms	Tightness of oedematous skin; abdominal discomfort	Tightness
Signs common to both	Swelling of lip(s)	
Discriminatory signs	None if confined to lips	None if confined to lips, but smaller urticarial weals around the mouth may also occur
Associated features	Urticaria may occur at other body sites. In the hereditary type, and in allergic reactions to allergens such as peanuts, other symptoms may occur; these include abdominal pain and vomiting, bronchospasm, laryngeal oedema, generalized urticaria, and anaphylaxis.	Discrete weals, sometimes with vesicles, may aris at other sites of contact; this process usually occurs with contact to proteins in cheese, eggs, etc.
Important tests	Enquire about ingestion of salicylates and other drugs which cause non-allergic histamine release from mast cells. Complement levels (C3, C4, C1-esterase inhibitor level), RAST, prick tests, drug history (immunological and non-immunological mechanisms); history of recent infections	Prick tests if required; radioallergosorbent test (RAST); contact urticaria testing

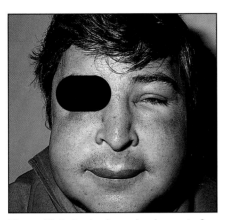

Figure 12.1 *Angioedema: involvement of face and eyelids as well as lips is uncommon in pure contact urticaria.*

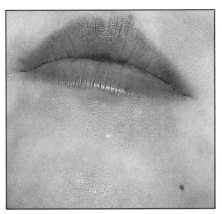

Figure 12.2 *Contact urticaria due to latex in a balloon. Reactions to rubber are usually due to chemicals in rubber manufacture, which cause a a delayed contact dermatitis, but latex itself may cause immediate contact urticaria. Some foods, such as avocado, banana, and chestnuts, may cause the same reaction in such patients.*

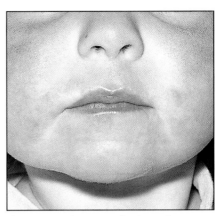

Figure 12.3 *Contact urticaria to cheese: one hand was also affected.*

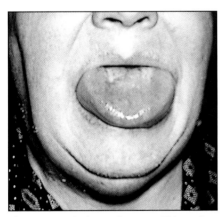

Figure 12.4 *Oedema of tongue. This patient had repeated episodes of tongue swelling but no involvement of any other site; the cause was contact urticaria due to a food flavouring .*

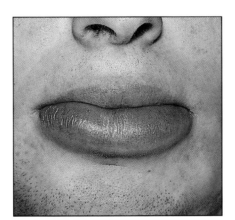

Figure 12.5 *Orofacial granulomatosis: this is a chronic, although initially variable disorder in which food allergies may sometimes be identified.*

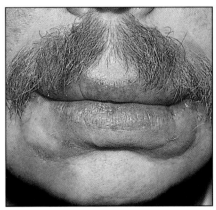

Figure 12.6 *Crohn's disease of the lip: this is usually less variable than orofacial granulomatosis, and with cobblestoned mucosal lesions.*

Further reading:
p. 20, p. 22, p. 100, p. 112.

References
Cicardi M, Agostoni A. Hereditary angioedema. *N Engl J Med* 1996; **334**:1666–7.
Donaldson VH. The challenge of hereditary angioneurotic edema. *N Engl J Med* 1983; **308**:1094–5.
Ellis CN (ed). Current management of urticaria and angioedema. Proceedings of a roundtable. *J Am Acad Dermatol* 1991; **25**:145–204.
Harvell J, Bason M, Maibach HI. Contact urticaria (immediate reaction syndrome). *Clinical Rev Allergy* 1992; **10**:303–23.

Ishii N, *et al*. Hereditary angioedema caused by a point mutation of exon 7 in the C1 inhibitor gene. *Br J Dermatol* 1996; **134**:731–3.
Nielsen EW, *et al*. Hereditary angioedema: new clinical observations and auto-immune screening, complement and kallikrein-kinin analysis. *J Int Med* 1996; **239**:119–30.
Williamson DM. Reticulate erythema: a prodrome of hereditary angioedema. *Br J Dermatol* 1979; **101**:548–52.

13 Infantile seborrhoeic eczema v. atopic eczema

Common presenting feature: widespread facial and truncal eczema.

Rationale for comparison: different prognosis and intensity of therapy necessary.

Other differential diagnoses: candidal infection; infantile psoriasis; irritant dermatitis; impetigo; scabies (p. 106).

Conclusion and key points: infantile seborrhoeic and atopic eczema are both common, and may both occur in the same child. Seborrhoeic eczema usually starts in the first few months of life, atopic eczema usually starting after the first few months. Confusion arises because the typical childhood flexural pattern of atopic eczema is preceded by a more diffuse facial and patchy truncal pattern. In early months, predominant scalp and flexural involvement, and well-defined scaling lesions, favour a diagnosis of seborrhoeic eczema. The best clinical discriminator is the general affect; children with extensive atopic eczema are uniformly itchy and miserable, while children with seborrhoeic dermatitis have an extensive rash but are considerably less upset by it than their parents are.

Comparative features		
Disorder	**Infantile seborrhoeic eczema**	**Infantile atopic eczema**
Age	Usually 1–6 months	Any, but mostly over six months
Sex	Either	
Family history	Non-specific	Usually positive for atopy
Sites	Scalp (usually initial site but often not inflammatory), face, nappy area, axillae, trunk	Face, trunk, limbs
Symptoms	Mild itch may occur, especially if there is secondary infection	Profound itch, disturbed sleep
Signs common to both	Eczematous rash on face, trunk, limb flexures	
Discriminatory signs	Lesions are generally sharply demarcated with yellowish greasy scale; cradle cap is usual. The infant is not greatly disturbed.	Lesions are more diffuse and with finer scaling or crusting. Marked itch and an overtly unhappy infant are typical.
Associated features	Preceding cradle cap is frequent	May be other signs of secondary infection, e.g. lymphadenopathy
Important tests	Bacteriology swabs to identify secondary infection (including yeasts)	Bacteriology swabs to identify secondary infection (typically staphylococcal). IgE level is raised in 80% of atopics and may be a useful support if there is diagnostic doubt.
Treatments	Mild topical steroids and anti-septic, anti-yeast agents (to eradicate *Pityrosporum ovale*) emollients	Emollients, topical corticosteroids, bandaging, oral antibiotics, oral antihistamines

Further reading:
p. 2, p. 28, p. 38, p. 122.

References
Kay J, *et al*. The prevalence of childhood atopic eczema in a general population. *J Am Acad Dermatol* 1994; **30**:35–9.
Podmore P, *et al*. Seborrhoeic eczema—a disease entity or a clinical variant of atopic eczema? *Br J Dermatol* 1986; **115**:341–50.McHenry PM, Williams HC, Bingham EA. Management of atopic eczema. Joint workshop of the British Association of Dermatologists and the research unit of the Royal College of Physicians of London. *BMJ* 1995; **310**:843–7.
Yates VM, *et al*. Early diagnosis of infantile seborrhoeic dermatitis and atopic dermatitis—clinical features. *Br J Dermatol* 1983; **108**:633–8.
Yates VM, *et al*. Early diagnosis of infantile seborrhoeic dermatitis and atopic dermatitis—total and specific IgE levels. *Br J Dermatol* 1983; **108**:639–45.

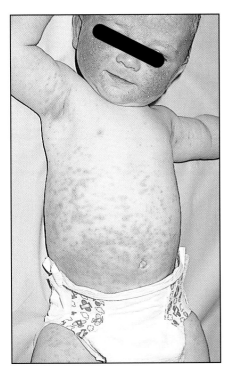

Figure 13.1
Infantile seborrhoeic dermatitis: there are widely scattered discrete and semi-confluent lesions, but the child is not unhappy (see also Fig. 61.2).

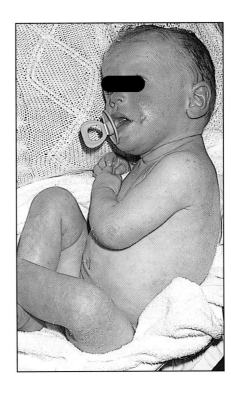

Figure 13.2
Infantile atopic dermatitis: there is more diffuse pinkness and fine scaling in an overtly miserable infant.

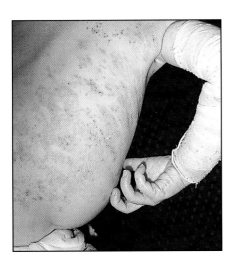

Figure 13.3 *Atopic dermatitis: the hallmark of this disorder is the presence of itch.*

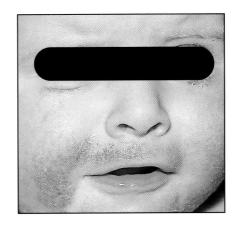

Figure 13.4
Infantile atopic dermatitis affecting the face.

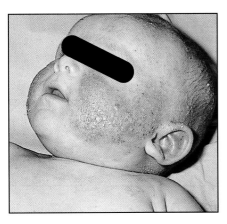

Figure 13.5
Infantile seborrhoeic dermatitis of the face: although this diagnosis is suggested by the rather greasy crusting, it is very difficult to differentiate it from atopic dermatitis by only viewing the face.

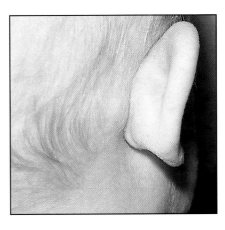

Figure 13.6 *Scalp involvement in the two disease processes can be difficult to differentiate: post-auricular lymphadenopathy is much more common in atopic than in seborrhoeic dermatitis.*

14 Seborrhoeic eczema v. rosacea

Common presenting feature: facial rash, which may be of 'butterfly' distribution affecting the cheeks.

Rationale for comparison: these two disorders are frequently confused but their treatments are different.

Other differential diagnoses: lupus erythematosus; contact dermatitis (to cosmetics or airborne allergens [p. 32]); photosensitivity (p. 32) or photoaggravated skin diseases.

Conclusion and key points: both disorders are commonly found and therefore may occur in the same individual. Facial seborrhoeic eczema usually affects the nasolabial creases and paranasal region in contrast to the mid-cheek and nasal distribution of rosacea; it is scaly rather than papulopustular, and is brownish rather than beefy-red in colour. Dandruff and scaling in the eyebrows are commonly associated with seborrhoeic eczema, while perioral involvement is more typical of rosacea.

Comparative features		
Disorder	**Seborrhoeic eczema**	**Rosacea**
Age	Mainly young adulthood, but any age from late teens	Usually middle-age but wide ranging
Sex	Either; more common in male	Either, female predominance
Family history	Non-specific	Nonspecific
Sites	Nasolabial and paranasal areas. Scaling may be present in eyebrows, scalp (especially marginal), ears, and postauricular creases. There may be scaling and erythema of the eyelid margin (blepharitis).	The nose, cheeks, forehead, and chin are typically affected. Perioral distribution (confusingly known as perioral dermatitis) is a variant, typically with a narrow zone of sparing around the lips. The eyelids are usually spared.
Symptoms	None, itch. Symptoms often provoked by heat and changes in humidity	None, itch, burning; may be aggravated by heat, sunlight, emotional stress
Signs common to both	Mid-facial erythema. Scaling may occur in rosacea but usually only in the older age group.	
Discriminatory signs	Brownish shade of red. Greasy scaling (common), or finer scaling of scalp. The site distribution as noted above is characteristic.	Beefier red colour. Papules, pustules, whiteheads (none are a feature of seborrhoeic eczema). Telangiectasia, especially nasal. Facial oedema may occur. Scaling is not a prominent feature but may occur at sites of old pustules.
Associated features	Diffuse (dandruff) or patchy scalp scaling. Seborrhoeic eczema may be present as scaly red patches at other sites (especially central chest or upper mid-back (in males) and axillae or groin flexures). Blepharitis causes itchy eyes.	Ocular rosacea (various symptoms, including grittiness, photophobia, excessive tears; objective signs include keratitis, conjunctivitis, corneal vascularization). Easy flushing. Rhinophyma and fixed telangiectasia may develop.
Important tests	None unless unusually extensive or associated with other infections or malaise. Seborrhoeic eczema is common in HIV infection.	None unless there is diagnostic doubt (especially to exclude lupus erythematosus)
Therapeutic implications	Best treated with an anti-yeast agent (e.g. an imidazole cream), alone or combined with a mild topical corticosteroid	Treat with topical or oral antibiotics (usually metronidazole topically, tetracyclines or erythromycin orally). Topical steroids may transiently suppress rosacea but tachyphylaxis and rebound flare are expected, leading to risk of steroid-induced telangiectasia.

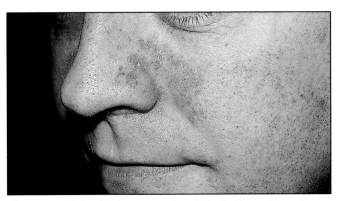

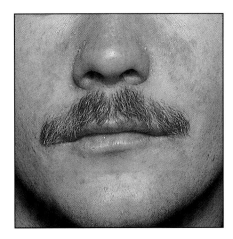

Figure 14.2
*Seborrhoeic
dermatitis: note the
distribution in a
'butterfly' pattern.*

Figure 14.1 *Seborrhoeic eczema: there is typical brownish erythema
and scaling in paranasal distribution.*

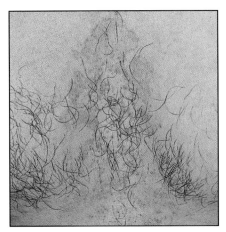

Figure 14.3 *Seborrhoeic dermatitis of
central chest, a useful discriminatory sign
when present (usually in male patients).*

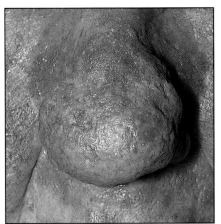

Figure 14.4 *Pustular lesions and
rhinophyma in rosacea.*

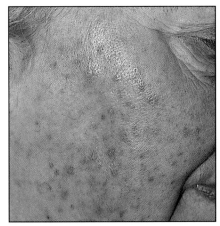

Figure 14.5 *Papular lesions of rosacea: the
discrete papules and overall extent are not
consistent with seborrhoeic dermatitis.*

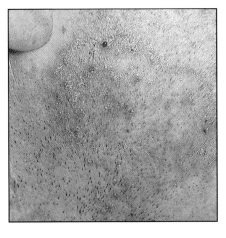

Figure 14.6 *Facial
tinea: erythema,
scaling, and pustules
may all occur but the
asymmetry and
marginal
accentuation should
allow easy
distinction from
rosacea or
seborrhoeic
dermatitis.*

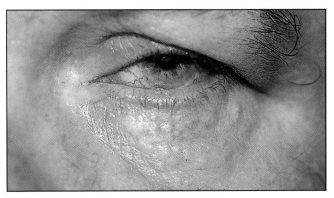

Figure 14.7 *A red eye due to rosacea: eye symptoms are common
but often non-specific.*

Further reading:
p. 2, p. 26, p. 30, p. 32, p. 38, p. 40.

References
Quarterman MJ, *et al.* Ocular rosacea. Signs, symptoms, and tear studies
  before and after treatment with doxycycline. *Arch Dermatol* 1997;
  133:49–54.
Rebora A. The red face: rosacea. *Clinics Dermatol* 1993; **11**:225–34.
Rhodes LE, Parslow RA, Ashworth J. Outcome of facial rashes with

non-specific histological features: a long term follow-up of 64 cases. *J
  Cutan Pathol* 1995; **22**:160–3.
Siberge S, Gawkrodger DJ. Rosacea, a study of clinical patterns, blood flow,
  and the role of demodex folliculorum. *J Am Acad Dermatol* 1992;
  26:590–3.
Wilkin JK. Rosacea. Pathophysiology and treatment. *Arch Dermatol* 1994;
  130:359–62.

15 Rosacea v. lupus erythematosus

Common presenting feature: facial rash, which typically affects the cheeks in a 'butterfly' distribution.

Rationale for comparison: there are important prognostic and therapeutic differences between these conditions, in particular the potential for scarring in discoid LE and the internal organ involvement of systemic lupus erythematosus.

Other differential diagnoses: eczemas; polymorphic light eruption; Jessner's lymphocytic dermatosis; photosensitivity disorders.

Conclusion and key points: patients with the butterfly rash of systemic LE virtually always have other symptoms to suggest the diagnosis. In a healthy patient, a butterfly rash is far more likely to be caused by rosacea. Discoid LE lesions are more discrete, and usually not associated with systemic disease, though they are one of the American Rheumatology Association criteria which may contribute to a diagnosis of systemic LE.

Comparative features		
Disorder	**Rosacea**	**Lupus erythematosus (LE)**
Age	Adult, especially middle-age	Systemic LE, mainly in young adults; discoid LE in adult (childhood cases rare)
Sex	Either	Systemic LE: marked female predominance of about 8:1 (F:M). Discoid LE ratio about 2:1 (F:M)
Family history	Non-specific	Occasionally positive
Sites	Mid-cheek, nasal	Systemic LE butterfly rash is mid-facial. Discoid LE lesions are generally more scattered.
Symptoms	None, itch, burning	None, itch
Signs common to both	Mid-facial erythematous rash	
Discriminatory signs	Erythematous papules, pustules, whiteheads. Lack of associated malaise or systemic symptoms	Absence of specific features of rosacea, sometimes tumid lesions; follicular keratotic plugs (tintack sign) and epidermal atrophy or frank scarring in discoid LE lesions. Follicular plugs in the concha are a useful sign but not specific. Scalp lesions of discoid LE often scar (see p. 6)
Associated features	Ocular rosacea	Other cutaneous features in systemic LE include photosensitivity, diffuse or scarring alopecia, nailfold changes. Systemic symptoms include malaise, arthralgia, and symptoms in the major organ systems (renal, cardiac, neuropsychiatric).
Important tests	None routinely; may require assessment of ocular rosacea	Serological proof of diagnosis and disease activity (ANA and others), skin biopsy and immunofluorescence, others as dictated by systemic symptoms (include haematological screen, renal function, markers of inflammation, other antibodies)

Further reading:

p. 6, p. 42, p. 44.

References

Kligman AM. Ocular rosacea. Current concepts and therapy. *Arch Dermatol* 1997; **133**:89–90.

Norris DA. Pathomechanisms of photosensitive lupus erythematosus. *J Invest Dermatol* 1993; **100**:58S–68S.

Rebora A, Drago F, Parodi A. May *Helicobacter pylori* be important for dermatologists? *Dermatology* 1995; **191**:6–8.

Sontheimer RD, Provost TT. Lupus erythematosus. In: Sontheimer RD, Provost TT (eds). *Cutaneous manifestations of rheumatic diseases*. Williams & Wilkins, Baltimore, 1996:1–71.

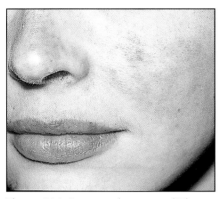

Figure 15.1 *Lupus erythematosus (LE) displaying the 'butterfly rash' seen in systemic LE.*

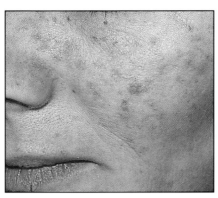

Figure 15.2 *Lupus erythematosus: this is a more papular rash than that of Fig. 15.1 but with the same distribution.*

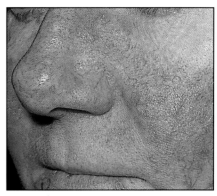

Figure 15.3 *Rosacea: this has a butterfly distribution similar to that seen in Fig. 15.1.*

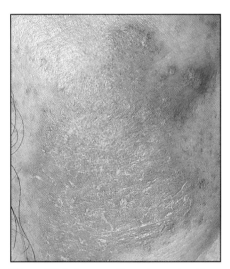

Figure 15.4 *Lupus erythematosus: tumid lesions in a patient with acute discoid LE (see also acute oedema due to rosacea and due to LE [Figs. 21.5 and 21.6]).*

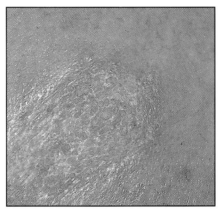

Figure 15.5 *Follicular keratotic plugs: these are a characteristic feature of discoid LE. Similar plugs occur in lichen sclerosus et atrophicus (see also Fig. 46.1).*

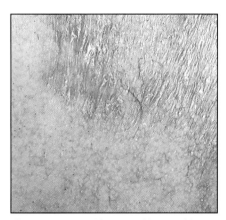

Figure 15.6 *Discoid LE: an older atrophic, telangiectatic and scarred lesion of discoid LE is seen.*

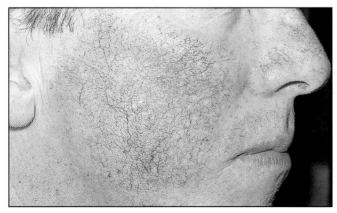

Figure 15.7 *Rosacea: there may be prominent telangiectasia, but this is more diffuse than in discoid LE (in which it is confined to discrete lesions) and is not accompanied by atrophy.*

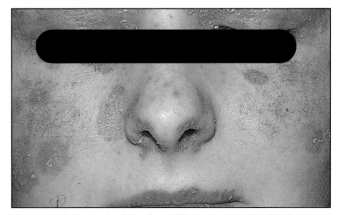

Figure 15.8 *Psoriasis of the face: this may mimic discoid LE, but lesions are usually present at other sites and the scalp margin is typically affected.*

Photosensitivity v. airborne contact dermatitis

Common presenting feature: an eczematous eruption affecting exposed sites.

Rationale for comparison: these disorders are easily confused as they have a similar site distribution and morphology. There are, however, different causes and thus different implications for prevention.

Other differential diagnoses: rosacea; other forms of contact dermatitis; seborrhoeic dermatitis; dermatomyositis; lupus erythematosus; photoaggravated rashes (e.g. some types of psoriasis and dermatitis); plant contact and photocontact reactions.

Conclusion and key points: airborne contact dermatitis (ACD) and photosensitivity can be very difficult to differen-tiate; both may worsen after outdoor activity. Some patterns of photosensitivity, e.g. solar urticaria or polymorphic light eruption, are most likely to be confused with rosacea or lupus erythematosus; most drug-induced photosensitivity is more dermatitic. The latter typically spares sun-shielded sites, e.g. skin creases and shaded areas under the nose, eyebrows, and chin. By contrast, ACD often preferentially affects skin creases, neck-line, and eyelids initially. However, both disorders may extend to affect the entire face and neck and may become impossible to differentiate without specialized tests. Idiopathic photosensitivity dermatitis (actinic reticuloid) mainly occurs in elderly men. Its cause is particularly difficult to resolve as there may be evidence of both contact sensitivities (positive patch tests), light sensitivity, and sometimes photocontact dermatitis (abnormal photosensitivity tests).

Comparative features		
Disorder	**Photosensitivity**	**Airborne contact dermatitis (ACD)**
Age	Any, depending on type, e.g: polymorphic light eruption (PLE). Typical onset is teenage/young adulthood; idiopathic photosensitivity dermatitis/actinic reticuloid pattern (PD/AR), and drug–induced. Onset is usually middle-aged/elderly	Any
Sex	Either (but different types affect the sexes preferentially, e.g. marked female predominance in PLE, male predominance in PD/AR)	Either
Family history	May be positive in PLE, but negative in most photosensitivity disorders	Negative
Sites	Any part of exposed skin. In early/acute eruption, spares shielded areas (skin creases, eyelids, below nose and chin)	Any part of exposed skin. In early cases, may affect creases and friction areas around neckline preferentially.
Symptoms	Itch	
Signs common to both	Diffuse eczematous rash affecting face and V of neck. Note that both disorders may progress to cause a confluent rash. A seasonal pattern is not a categorical distinguishing factor, as airborne contact dermatitis may be due to airborne plant products, whereas some types of photosensitivity cause perennial symptoms.	
Discriminatory signs	Initial sparing of skin creases and shaded areas (see above)	Preferential involvement of skin creases
Associated features	Dorsum of hands and forearms frequently affected. Other features depend on the cause, e.g. an urticarial component in polymorphic light eruption, contact allergies in photosensitivity dermatitis.	Other exposed areas are often affected.
Important tests	Phototest, patch test, photopatch test, antinuclear antibody (and anti-Ro [=SSA] plus anti-LA [=SSB] antibodies for subacute cutaneous LE). Porphyrin screen may be indicated (see p. 74)	
Potential identifiable causes	Drug causes of photosensitivity: commonest are thiazides, non-steroidal anti-inflammatory drugs, sulphonamides, quinine, amiodarone, chlorpromazine	Airborne allergens are frequently plant materials, e.g. Balsams, fragrances (including household plants, air fresheners, hair sprays), compositae (daisy family). Also consider phosphorus sequisulphide in red match heads and the striking surface of safety match-boxes.

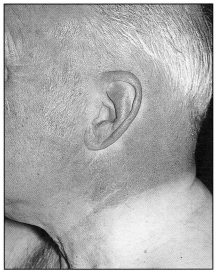

Figure 16.1 *Photosensitivity (drug-induced): this shows cut-off at neck-line.*

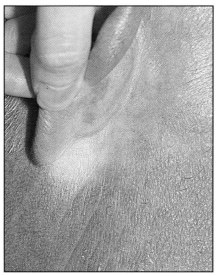

Figure 16.2 *Photosensitivity (drug-induced): retro-auricular sparing is shown.*

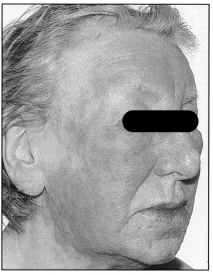

Figure 16.3 *Photosensitivity: there is similar sparing under the frontal hair margin in drug-induced photosensitivity rash.*

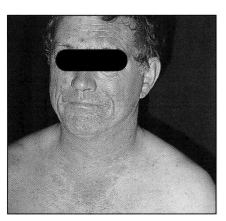

Figure 16.4
Airborne contact dermatitis due to Balsam in pine wood, with distribution simulating that of a photosensivity eruption.

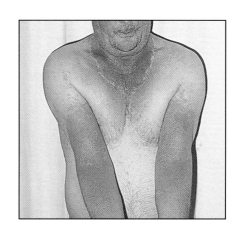

Figure 16.5
Airborne contact dermatitis simulating photosensitivity rash.

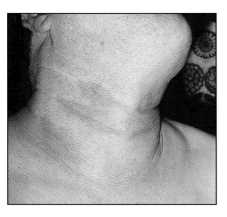

Figure 16.6
Airborne contact dermatitis due to Balsam, preferentially affecting the sweaty (and relatively less light exposed) skin creases of the neck.

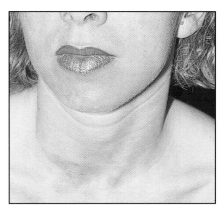

Figure 16.7 *Contact allergy due to nail varnish. This typically affects the face and neck with a streaky pattern which may simulate that of photosensitivity rash or airborne contact dermatitis.*

Further reading:
p. 22, p. 24, p. 28, p. 30, p. 38, p. 40, p. 42, p. 76.

References
Dooms-Goossens A, *et al*. Contact dermatitis caused by airborne agents. *J Am Acad Dermatol* 1986; **15**:1–10.
Gonzalez E, Gonzalez S. Drug photosensitivity, idiopathic photodermatoses, and sunscreens. *J Am Acad Dermatol* 1996; **35**:871–5.
Gould JW, Mercurio MG, Elmets CA. Cutaneous photosensitivity diseases induced by exogenous agents. *J Am Acad Dermatol* 1995; **33**:551–73.
Roelandts R. Chronic actinic dermatitis. *J Am Acad Dermatol* 1993; **28**:240–9.

17 Acne v. pseudofolliculitis

Common presenting feature: papular and pustular lesions in the beard area.

Rationale for comparison: pseudofolliculitis is often confused with acne. Consequently, affected men may be prescribed inappropriate prolonged antibiotic therapy.

Other differential diagnoses: true folliculitis (including herpes simplex, staphylococcal, Gram-negative and pityrosporum folliculitis); carbuncles; epidermoid cysts.

Conclusion and key points: pseudofolliculitis is a mechanical problem of ingrowing curved hairs. It is not caused by increased sebum production and follicular occlusion. It can usually be differentiated from acne by visualizing hairs curving into the pustules, and by the fact that it is limited to the beard area. However, it is common in young men and may therefore coexist with acne in later teenage years. Pseudofolliculitis does not respond to anti-inflammatory medication but can be treated in milder cases by mechanical removal of ingrowing hairs. In more extensive cases, the best treatment is to grow a beard.

Comparative features		
Disorder	**Acne**	**Pseudofolliculitis**
Age	Mostly early teens to 20s	Late teens onward
Sex	Either	Male
Family history	May be positive	Non-specific
Sites	Beard area and other facial and upper truncal sites	Confined to beard area on the face (may also occur on thighs or abdomen)
Symptoms	None, tenderness	
Signs common to both	Papules and pustules in beard area, sometimes deeper nodules also	
Discriminatory signs	Other types of acne lesions, on the face or at other sites; these include open and closed comedones, and greasy skin. Note that these may coexist with pseudofolliculitis in some individuals (usually late teens or older).	Visible ingrowing hairs, which can be carefully extracted with a needle (Figs 17.3, and 17.4). No response to acne therapy
Associated features		Usually affects individuals with curly or wavy hair, and is particularly common in African–Caribbean races
Important tests	None	
Treatment	Numerous topical anti-comedonal and anti-inflammatory agents, oral antibiotics, isotretinoin	Mechanical; lift out ingrowing hairs with needle, avoid close shaving, grow beard. Occasionally, excision of lesions if large and persistent

Further reading:
p. 36, p. 88.

References
Cunliffe WJ. *Acne*. Martin Dunitz, London, 1989
Healy E, Simpson N. Acne vulgaris. *BMJ* 1994; **308**:831–3.

Kaminer MS, Gilchrest BA. The many faces of acne. *J Am Acad Dermatol* 1995; **32**:S6–14.

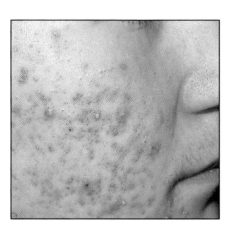

Figure 17.1 *Acne in the beard area with scarring and pustules. Note lesions beyond the area of beard hairs (pseudofolliculitis is confined to the area of beard hair growth).*

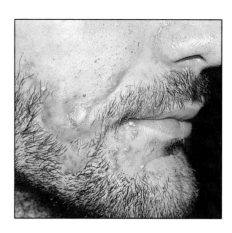

Figure 17.2 *Cystic acne: lesions of this size can occur in pseudofolliculitis (see Fig. 17.5), but are very unusual.*

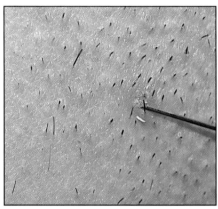

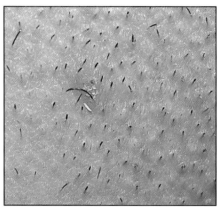

Figures 17.3 and 17.4 *Pseudofolliculitis, demonstrating an ingrowing hair being lifted out of the skin.*

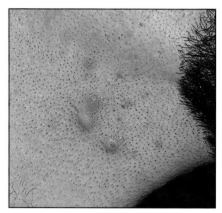

Figure 17.5 *Pseudofolliculitis: larger nodules may be a feature in occasional cases.*

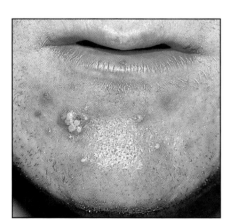

Figure 17.6 *Gram-negative folliculitis is usually more acute and more uniformly pustular than true acne or pseudofolliculitis.*

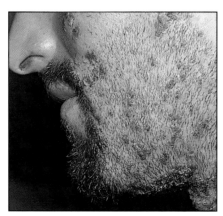

Figure 17.7 *Impetigo due to staphylococci in the beard area is more rapidly progressive and extensive: note that herpes simplex folliculitis may be very similar to this.*

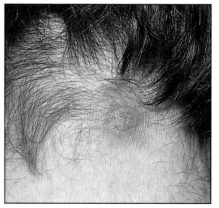

Figure 17.8 *Carbuncle (boil): this is usually solitary and more acutely tender than acne or pseudofolliculitis.*

18 Acne v. tuberous sclerosis (adenoma sebaceum)

Common presenting feature: skin-coloured or erythematous mid-facial papules.

Rationale for comparison: milder, especially sporadic, cases of adenoma sebaceum may not present until teenage years. Accurate diagnosis is essential for genetic counselling, and avoids unnecessary treatment for acne.

Other differential diagnoses: naevi; plane warts; telangiectasia; neurofibromas; cysts; various follicular neoplasia (especially syringomas, trichoepitheliomas); multiple endocrine neoplasia type 1.

Conclusion and key points: adenoma sebaceum (angiofibromas), the facial lesion of tuberous sclerosis, may be confused with therapy-resistant acne. However, patients with adenoma sebaceum do not have the range of lesions typical of acne; comedones, pustules, and deeper nodules are not a feature of tuberous sclerosis. Lesions of various types at other body sites, including depigmented 'ash-leaf' patches, collagenomas, and periungual fibromas, may confirm the diagnosis of tuberous sclerosis. Facial angiofibromas are also common in multiple endocrine neoplasia, type 1, but without other signs of tuberous sclerosis. Tuberous sclerosis is a potentially severe inherited condition; it has autosomal dominant inheritance but sporadic cases occur, and such patients require genetic counselling about the potential risks to their future offspring.

Comparative features		
Disorder	**Acne**	**Adenoma sebaceum**
Age	Teens to 20s	May present at any age; mild or sporadic cases may present in teens
Sex	Either	
Family history	Non-specific	Usually positive (autosomal dominant) but up to 50% of cases may arise as new mutations
Sites	Face; may affect neck, back, chest	Usually predominantly mid-face (nasal and paranasal)
Symptoms	None, tenderness	None
Signs common to both	Skin coloured or erythematous papules	
Discriminatory signs	Other lesions in the acne spectrum, such as comedones, pustules, and deeper nodules. Acne at other body sites, especially shoulders/upper trunk, is common.	The facial angiofibromas are skin-coloured to red and typically monomorphic. Diagnostic skin lesions at other sites (usually truncal) include pale oval shaped 'ash-leaf' macules, best seen using Wood's light examination, and collagenomas, which are known as 'shagreen patches'. Multiple peri-ungual fibromas may be present.
Associated features	None	Various internal manifestations, especially neurological lesions (cortical tubers, subependymal nodules), which may cause epilepsy or mental retardation. Other internal manifestations include retinal (astrocytomas and hamartomas), cardiac (rhabdomyoma), renal (cysts, angiomyolipoma), and dental lesions (enamel pits, gingival fibromas).
Important tests	None	Identification of internal involvement, especially cerebral imaging

Further reading:
p. 34, p. 88.

References
Hunt A. Tuberous sclerosis: a survey of 97 cases. II. Physical findings. *Devel Med Child Neurol* 1983; **25**:350–2.
Moss C, Savin J. *Dermatology and the new genetics.* Blackwell Science, Oxford, 1995.

Roach ES, Delgado MR. Tuberous sclerosis. *Dermatol Clinics* 1995; **13**:151–61.
Sykes NL, Webster GF. Acne: a review of optimum treatment. *Drugs* 1994; **48**:59–70.

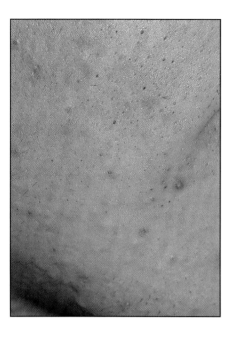

Figure 18.1
Comedones: these are a feature of true acne which do not occur in tuberous sclerosis.

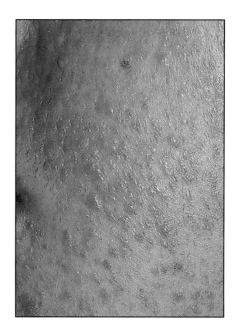

Figure 18.2
Tuberous sclerosis: there are relatively monomorphic papular lesions present.

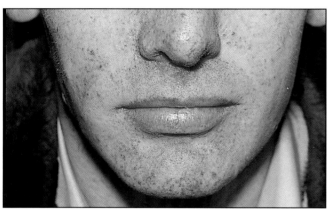

Figure 18.3 *Tuberous sclerosis: small vascular lesions are present (angiofibromas, or adenoma sebaceum).*

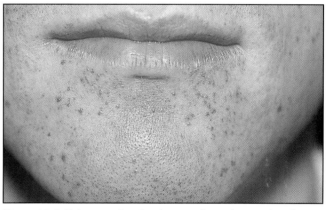

Figure 18.4 *Tuberous sclerosis: close-up of vascular papules of adenoma sebaceum which developed in teenage years and were treated as acne.*

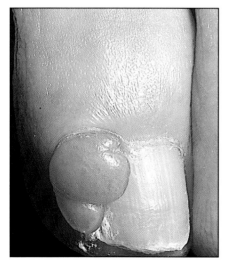

Figure 18.5
Periungual fibroma: this is a useful confirmatory sign of tuberous sclerosis. Note, however, that solitary lesions can occur as a sporadic finding without systemic significance. (See also Fig. 89.3.)

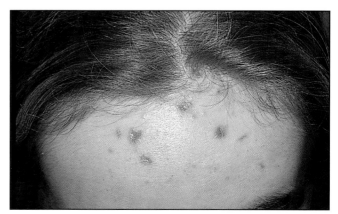

Figure 18.6 *Acne excoriée: this is a pattern of acne which is dominated by 'picked' spots, and which causes diagnostic confusion due to the relative lack of typical acne lesions.*

19 Eyelid contact dermatitis v. other eyelid eczemas

Common presenting feature: itch, scaling, and erythema of eyelids.

Rationale for comparison: these disorders may be very difficult to differentiate clinically, but there are different therapeutic implications of allergen avoidance (see Table) in cases of contact dermatitis.

Other differential diagnoses: other inflammatory dermatoses affecting eyelids (e.g. discoid lupus erythematosus, dermatomyositis, rosacea blepharitis); localized eyelid lesions (e.g. syringomas).

Conclusion and key points: the main differential diagnoses are contact, atopic, and seborrhoeic dermatitis of eyelids. Potential allergens can sometimes be determined by the clinical history. The age of onset may be helpful; atopic dermatitis affecting eyelids is most common in childhood, but may persist into adult life, while contact or seborrhoeic dermatitis usually develops for the first time in adult years. In patients with atopic or seborrhoeic dermatitis of the eyelids, there are usually features of the underlying disorder at other sites (e.g. flexural dermatitis in atopics, dandruff or seborrhoeic dermatitis of face or chest in patients with eyelid seborrhoeic blepharitis). In some cases, distinguishing between these disorders can be very difficult, and patch testing may be helpful. Additionally, contact dermatitis may complicate the other disorders if patients become allergic to eyedrops or ointments (see Table). It is particularly difficult to identify an avoidable cause in patients with seasonal eyelid eczema, which is presumably caused by airborne plant pollens or fragrances.

Comparative features		
Disorder	**Contact allergy, eyelid**	**Other eyelid dermatitis (atopic, seborrhoeic)**
Age	Adult	Atopic eyelid dermatitis usually starts in early childhood. Seborrhoeic blepharitis is often first manifest in teens or early adult years.
Sex	Female predominance, due to the higher frequency of perfume use and nickel allergy in women	Either
Family history	Nonspecific	May be positive
Sites	The specific eyelid sites may vary with cause. Most are diffuse, but in the early stages the distribution may reflect sites of application of the contact allergen (e.g. reactions to mascara or eyelash adhesives affect the lid margin; eyedrop reactions tend to affect the corners of the eyes).	Atopic dermatitis usually shows diffuse involvement, seborrhoeic dermatitis affects the eyelid margin (blepharitis).
Symptoms	Itch, burning	
Signs common to both	Erythema, scaling of eyelids	
Discriminatory signs	There are no specific physical signs to diagnose contact dermatitis of eyelids, although lack of evidence for atopic or seborrhoeic dermatitis is a useful negative finding. The history may be specifically related to direct application of certain products, or relate to specific seasons (airborne plant allergies).	May be typical atopic facies with Dennie–Morgan fold in lower eyelid skin. Seborrhoeic blepharitis tends to be more crusted and affects margin of eyelids. Note that presence of atopy does not preclude a contact allergy, especially in older children or adults
Associated features	Depends on cause. Features or history of cosmetic or nickel allergies are particularly likely to be relevant.	Atopic: facial and flexural dermatitis, asthma, hayfever, rhinitis Seborrhoeic: facial rash (p.28), dandruff, marginal scalp scaling, involvement of central chest or back
Important tests	Patch testing (see table of causes of likely allergens)	Elevated IgE level supports a diagnosis of atopy, RAST to house dust mite may be helpful. Patch tests may be indicated, especially in atopics with eyelid involvement out of proportion to other sites.

Causes of contact dermatitis of eyelids	
Cosmetics	Especially due to fragrance, colophony resin (e.g. mascara), and preservative components
Nail products	Nail varnish, glues
Airborne agents	Balsams/fragrances (from plants, sprays etc.), chemicals in match heads (phosphorus sequisulphide), latex, formaldehyde, epoxy resin vapour
Contact lens agents	Especially preservatives, e.g. thiomersal, benzalkonium chloride
Ophthalmic drugs	As for contact lens solutions, also antibiotics (e.g. neomycin) and other active drugs
Others	Nickel, plant materials

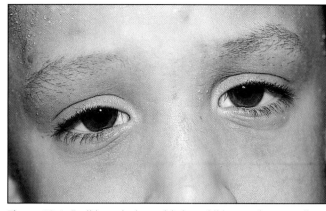

Figure 19.1 *Eyelid atopic dermatitis in a child: note the generally dry skin and prominent eyelid crease line (Dennie–Morgan fold).*

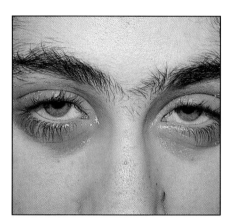

Figure 19.2 *Eyelid atopic dermatitis in an adult; this is a relatively frequent problem site in individuals with atopic dermatitis persisting into adult years.*

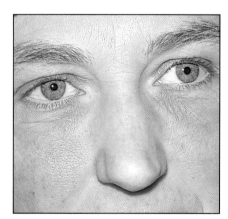

Figure 19.3 *Contact dermatitis of eyelids; This disorder gives patch test reactions to fragrance materials and a preservative agent commonly used in cosmetics.*

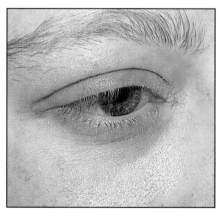

Figure 19.4 *Seborrhoeic blepharitis: a history of dandruff is frequent, and symptoms are often worst after being asleep overnight.*

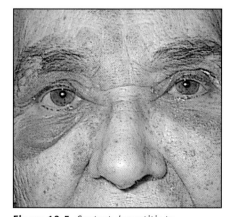

Figure 19.5 *Contact dermatitis to benzalkonium chloride, a preservative in eyedrops.*

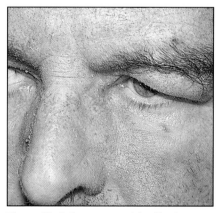

Figure 19.6 *Dermatomyositis affecting eyelids; the rash may appear somewhat eczematous but typically has a purplish or violaceous colour ('heliotrope rash').*

Further reading:
p. 22, p. 28, p. 32, p. 42, p. 76.

References
Cox NH. Allergy to benzalkonium hydrochloride simulating dermato myositis. *Contact Dermatitis* 1994; **31**:50.

Fisher AA. *Contact dermatitis*, 3rd edn. Philadelphia, Lea & Febiger, 1986:78–81.

Mannis MJ, Macsai MS, Huntley AC. *Eye and skin disease*. Lippincott–Raven, Philadelphia, 1996:149–74.

20 Eczema v. actinic keratoses

Common presenting feature: erythematous scaly areas.

Rationale for comparison: a common cause of diagnostic confusion in the older age-group, but different therapeutic implications.

Other differential diagnoses: discoid lupus erythematosus; certain basal cell carcinomas; Bowen's disease; nodular elastoidosis (Favre–Racouchot syndrome).

Conclusion and key points: discrete and overtly keratotic

actinic (solar) keratoses should not be confused with eczema, but the flatter and more telangiectatic versions are often mistakenly treated as eczema or unspecified inflammation. However, it is uncommon for discrete localized patches of facial eczema to occur for the first time in elderly patients. The more discrete nature, fixed position, and minimal symptoms, are the important diagnostic points for this type of actinic keratosis. In patients with several lesions the whole affected area feels rough and spiky. Actinic keratoses are often more easily felt than seen.

Comparative features		
Disorder	**Eczema**	**Actinic keratoses**
Age	Any	Middle-age, elderly
Sex	Either	
Family history	Non-specific	
Sites	Any	Chronically sun-exposed sites such as forehead, temples, bald scalp, nose, and ears
Symptoms	Itch	None, minor irritation
Signs common to both	Erythematous scaly areas, crusting	
Discriminatory signs	Fine scale, more diffuse erythematous background, severity and sites vary with time	More discrete and harder keratotic surface; lesions are typically more easily felt than seen. Some may be telangiectatic but do not have the diffuse erythema of an eczematous process; their fixed position (usually on forehead or temples) is also more suggestive of actinic keratosis.
Associated features	There may be eczema at other sites.	Other signs of solar damage, e.g. elastosis, cheilitis, more discrete keratoses of ears, scalp, dorsal surface of hands
Important tests	Patch testing may be required if a contact dermatitis is suspected.	Biopsy is required if there is concern about malignancy: progression to squamous cell carcinoma has been estimated to occur in 1/1000 actinic keratoses.

Further reading:
p. 20, p. 22, p. 32, p. 42, p. 54, pp. 74–78, p. 154.

References
Goette DK. Topical chemotherapy with 5-fluorouracil. A review. *J Am Acad Dermatol* 1981; **4**:633–49.
Sober AJ, Burstein JM. Precursors to skin cancer. *Cancer* 1995; **75**(Suppl 2): 645–50.

Thompson SC, *et al.* Reduction of solar keratoses by regular sunscreen use. *N Engl J Med* 1993; **329**:1147–9.

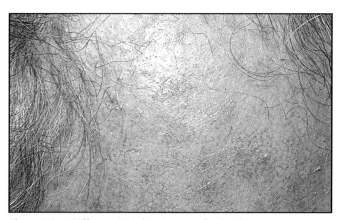

Figure 20.1 *Diffuse actinic keratoses on forehead.*

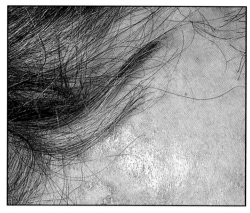

Figure 20.2 *Virtually flat actinic keratosis on the temple: this type of lesion is much more apparent from palpation than from visual examination only.*

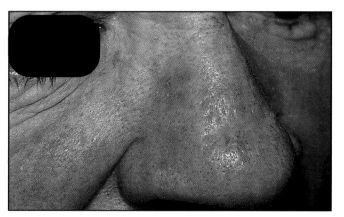

Figure 20.3 *Actinic keratoses on the nose, a pattern that may simulate that of seborrhoeic dermatitis.*

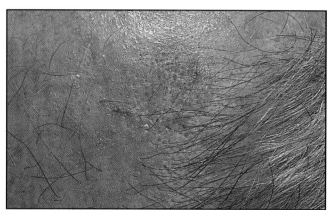

Figure 20.4 *Actinic keratinosis: prominent follicles in a flat actinic keratosis are seen.*

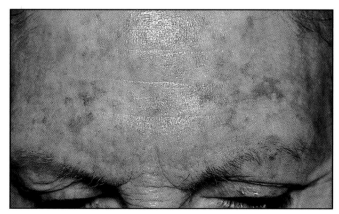

Figure 20.5 *Telangiectatic flat actinic keratoses: these often cause diagnostic problems.*

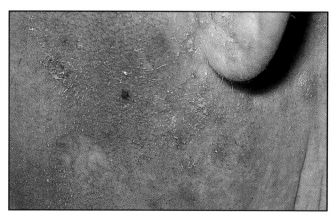

Figure 20.6 *Actinic keratoses on a background of solar damage (and previous radiotherapy for squamous cell carcinoma) on the cheek (same patient as in Fig. 27.5).*

21 Acute eczema v. erysipelas/cellulitis in adults

Common presenting feature: acute facial erythema.

Rationale for comparison: there are important therapeutic differences between these two disorders.

Other differential diagnoses: acute onset rosacea; herpes zoster; occasionally, lupus erythematosus, dermatomyositis.

Conclusion and key points: these acute eruptions can be difficult to differentiate. Erysipelas is usually more localized and demarcated than acute eczemas, and is not initially scaly, though it may desquamate in the regressing phase. Tenderness is the typical symptom of erysipelas, usually associated with significant malaise and pyrexia. Acute eczema is more itchy than tender, and facial swelling and weeping or crusting may be prominent features.

Comparative features

Disorder	Acute eczema	Erysipelas/cellulitis
Age	Any	Mostly middle-aged, elderly
Sex	Either	
Family history	Non-specific	
Sites	Any part of face; often includes or preferentially affects periorbital skin	Usually mid-facial, especially cheeks
Symptoms	Itch, discomfort	Tenderness, itch, burning (and general malaise, fever)
Signs common to both	Acute onset facial erythema +/– oedema, occasionally blisters and crusting	
Discriminatory signs	Diffuse facial involvement; scaling; may be small blisters	Sharp demarcation, beefy red colour, hot to touch, oedematous. Blisters are less common but often large if they do occur, and may be followed by skin necrosis.
Associated features	May be a history of more localized preceding eczema, or of a likely contact allergen (which may be a direct contact or airborne pattern, see p.32 and p.38)	Systemic features; malaise and pyrexia. There is occasionally a skin break at the portal of entry (if recurrent and unilateral, consider pre-auricular sinus).
Important tests	Patch testing to the European standard battery and other likely allergens (as for eyelids, p.38) should be performed but delayed until after the acute phase. Hair dye reactions typically affect the face and are characteristically severe. Bacteriology may be required as secondary infection is common in acute eczema.	Bacteriology if any blister or apparent portal of entry visible; antistreptolysin-O titre, anti-DN-ase B, markers of acute inflammation (erythrocyte sedimentation rate, C-reactive protein)
Paediatric equivalents	Acute facial dermatitis is usually of the atopic or seborrhoeic type (p.26) rather than the acute contact dermatitis with secondary staphylococcal infection.	Acute facial cellulitis is usually due to *Haemophilus* rather than *Streptococcus*.

Further reading:
p. 22, p. 24, pp. 28–32, p. 38, p. 76, p. 168.

References
Cox NH, Knowles MA, Porteus ID. Preseptal cellulitis and facial erysipelas due to *Moraxella* species. *Clin Exp Dermatol* 1994; **19**:321–3.

Jackson K, Baker SR. Periorbital cellulitis. *Head and Neck Surg* 1987; **9**:227–34.
Sachs MK. Cutaneous cellulitis. *Arch Dermatol* 1991; **127**:493–6.

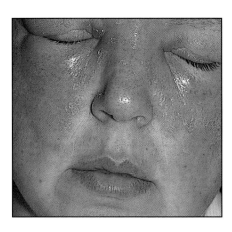

Figure 21.1
Erysipelas: there is a typical mid-facial distribution, with beefy-red erythema and facial swelling.

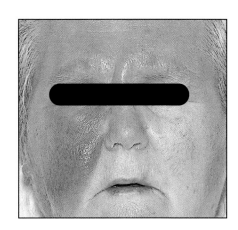

Figure 21.2
Erysipelas: the appearance is similar to that in Fig. 21.1 but shows less symmetry.

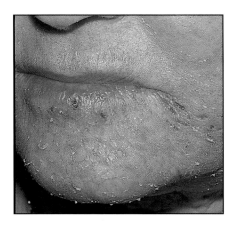

Figure 21.3 *Acute facial eczema: there is diffuse erythema and a marked scaling component.*

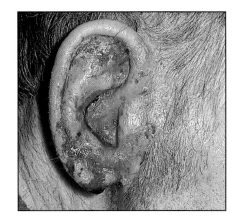

Figure 21.4 *Contact dermatitis to neomycin in eardrops: this may simulate a worsening cellulitis, but is scaly or crusted rather than primarily oedematous.*

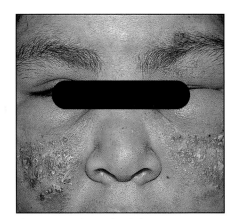

Figure 21.5 *Systemic LE: in very acute cases, the appearance may simulate that of a cellulitis.*

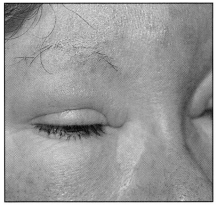

Figure 21.6 *Rosacea: this may present as facial oedema with a few typical papules and pustules (see also p. 30).*

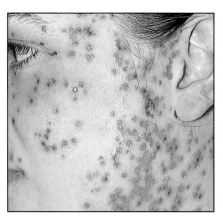

Figure 21.7 *Eczema herpeticum: herpes simplex in an atopic patient may be confused with cellulitis but the discrete umbilicated lesions are typical.*

22 Scleroderma/CREST syndrome v. hereditary haemorrhagic telangiectasia

Common presenting feature: facial telangiectases.

Rationale for comparison: there are some cutaneous similarities but different systemic implications.

Other differential diagnoses: spider naevi; solar telangiectasia; rosacea; ataxia telangiectasia; generalized essential telangiectasia; steroid-induced skin atrophy; unilateral naevoid telangiectasia.

Conclusion and key points: telangiectases of scleroderma spectrum disorders may be indistinguishable from those of hereditary haemorrhagic telangiectasia (HHT), though lesions on the lips, tongue, or nail-bed suggest HHT. Mat-like telangiectases, made up of multiple small vessels with an overall size of 2–20 mm, are more common in scleroderma and CREST (calcinosis, Raynaud's phenomenon, oesophageal dysmotility, sclerodactyly, telangiectasia) than in HHT. Other skin features, such as sclerosis, sclerodactyly, nailfold changes (ragged cuticles, dilated capillary loops), and radial furrows around the mouth, or restricted mouth opening, all favour scleroderma or CREST. Internal manifestations are different, and are listed in 'Comparative features'.

Comparative features		
Disorder	**Scleroderma/CREST**	**Hereditary haemorrhagic telangiectasia (HHT)**
Age	Any age but mostly adults	Mostly have lesions in teens but may show no symptoms
Sex	Either, mainly female	Either
Family history	Occasionally positive	Positive (autosomal dominant) but not always symptomatic
Sites	Telangiectasia mainly on cheeks and nose	Any part of face, usually including mucous membranes of lips, tongue, conjunctiva
Symptoms	Related to sclerosis rather than telangiectasia. Symptoms include Raynaud's phenomenon, cold hands (see p. 148), tightness of skin, pain of digital infarcts etc.	Epistaxis is most common. If patients with HHT develop malaise, fever, and respiratory or cerebral symptoms which are not due to anaemia, an arteriovenous shunt should be considered.
Signs common to both	Mid-facial telangiectasia (punctate and short linear lesions)	
Discriminatory signs	The telangiectases are not typically mucosal. Other cutaneous signs include sclerotic changes (sclerosis, especially sclerodactyly; radial furrows around mouth and limited mouth opening) and nailfold changes (elongated cuticles, sclerosis, and large capillary loops).	Mucosal involvement (buccal and tongue); telangiectasia of fingers occurs but without sclerotic changes (this may occur in early scleroderma also); nailbed telangiectases, finger clubbing (in patients with a pulmonary arteriovenous shunt)
Systemic features	Most organs may be affected. Most frequent and significant are oesophageal motility disorder, restrictive lung deficit, renal disease, calcified foci	Bleeding, especially epistaxis, causing anaemia. Arteriovenous shunts in lungs have potential risk of septic emboli.
Important tests	Assessment of internal disease	

Further reading:
p. 28, p. 30, p. 148.

References
Hodgson CH, *et al*. Hereditary haemorrhagic telangiectasia and pulmonary arteriovenous fistulae. *N Engl J Med* 1959; **261**:625–36.
Peery WH. Clinical spectrum of hereditary haemorrhagic telangiectasia (Osler–Weber–Rendu disease). *Am J Med* 1987;**82**:989–97.

Perez MI, Kohn SR. Systemic sclerosis. *J Am Acad Dermatol* 1993; **28**:525–47.
Porteus ME, Burn J, Proctor SJ. Hereditary haemorrhagic telangiectasia. A clinical analysis. *J Med Genet* 1992; **29**:527–30.
Reilly PG, Nostrant TT. Clinical manifestations of hereditary haemorrhagic telangiectasia. *Am J Gastroenterol* 1984; **79**:363–7.

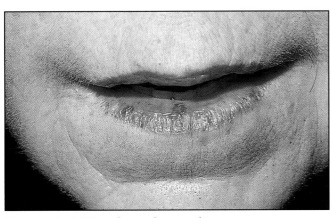

Figure 22.1 *CREST syndrome: there are short, tortuous telangiectases on the lips.*

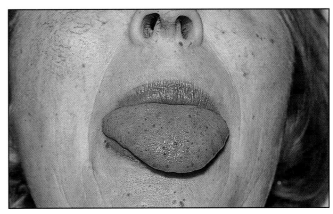

Figure 22.2 *Haemorrhagic telangiectasia of face and tongue: telangiectases are more punctate than in Fig. 22.1.*

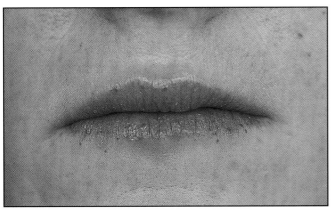

Figure 22.3 *Lip lesions in haemorrhagic telangiectasia : note absence of perioral 'radial furrowing' which may occur in scleroderma.*

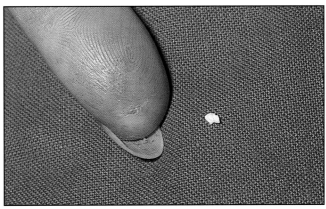

Figure 22.4 *Sclerodactyly and extruded calcified nodule in a patient with CREST.*

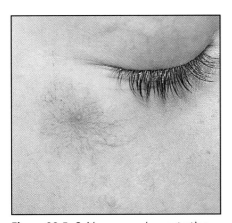

Figure 22.5 *Spider naevus demonstrating radiating telangiectasia: this pattern is not a feature of HHT or of scleroderma and CREST.*

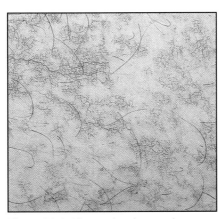

Figure 22.6 *Linear telangiectases in a patient with essential telangiectasia: vessels in rosacea, corticosteroid atrophy, and solar damage are less florid but have a similar morphology.*

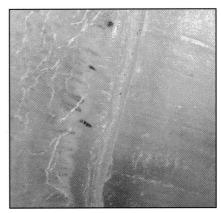

Figure 22.7 *Nailfold abnormalities of scleroderma and CREST syndrome.*

23 Nodular basal cell carcinoma v. intradermal naevus

Common presenting feature: pale or skin-coloured dome-shaped nodule, which may have visible surface telangiectasia.

Rationale for comparison: there are important treatment and follow-up differences. Benign naevi do not require intervention, but basal cell carcinoma should be removed.

Other differential diagnoses: solitary neurofibroma; sebaceous hyperplasia (p. 48); skin appendage neoplasia; cysts (p. 50); leiomyoma.

Conclusion and key points: most of the confusion between basal cell carcinoma (BCC) and naevi arises with relatively pale lesions, but pigmented BCC can also cause diagnostic problems. BCCs are typically more translucent and grey in colour than melanocytic naevi; this is often best appreciated if the skin is stretched under a good light. Non-pigmented intradermal naevi—the older type typically seen on the face—are covered by normal epidermis and therefore appear white or skin-coloured. Telangiectasia may be visible in either diagnosis but is usually more prominent in BCC. Intact follicles may be seen in either, but are usually destroyed in BCC, and hairs localized to the lesion are typical of intradermal naevi. However, the morphology of these two disorders may appear identical and the history is often the important differentiating feature; lesions which have been apparent and unchanging for several years are unlikely to be neoplastic.

Comparative features		
Disorder	**Nodular basal cell carcinoma (BCC)**	**Old intradermal naevus**
Age	Middle-age, elderly	Adulthood, but some pigment is normal in younger adult intradermal naevi
Sex	Either	
Family history	Non-specific	
Sites	Any area of face. Some sites, e.g. junction of cheek with ala nasi, are common to both. Either disorder may occur at other body sites but most diagnostic confusion applies to facial lesions.	
Symptoms	None; sometimes crusting. Lesions typically appear 1–2 years before patients attend.	None. Lesions typically appear 5–10 years before patients attend.
Signs common to both	Pale, smooth, dome-shaped nodule, may have surface telangiectasia	
Discriminatory signs	Usually solitary. Greyer, or pearly, colour compared with naevi (most easily visualized if the skin is stretched under a good light); surface telangiectases usually prominent. If pigmented, usually large dark grey–black blocks of pigment present. May have umbilicated surface. Usually loss of hairs if in a hair-bearing area, but follicles may be preserved in some BCCs. Size progressively increases, eventually causing ulceration and crusting	Fine 'dusting' of brown pigment. More white than grey in colour, finer telangiectases; may have hairs or visible follicular orifices. Multiple similar lesions are common.
Associated features	None	Often other naevi apparent
Important tests	Excision biopsy and histology	None

Further reading:
p. 12, p. 50, p. 86, p. 152, p. 156, p. 160, p. 162.

References
Cox NH. Basal cell carcinoma in young adults. *Br J Dermatol* 1992; **127**:26–9.

Goldberg LH. Basal cell carcinoma. *Lancet* 1996; **347**:663–7.
Randle HW. Basal cell carcinoma: identification and treatment of the high risk patient. *Dermatol Surg* 1996; **22**:255–61.

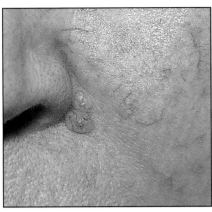

Figure 23.1 *Basal cell carcinoma (BCC) (lower lesion) and naevus (upper lesion) at a typical site for either disorder, demonstrating how similar they can appear.*

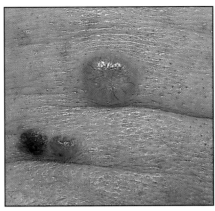

Figure 23.2 *Forehead lesions: the larger nodule is a BCC; the smaller ones are pigmented seborrhoeic keratosis (left) and melanocytic naevus (right).*

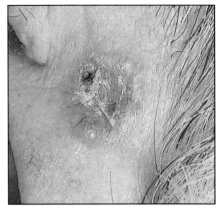

Figure 23.3 *Basal cell carcinoma: a later lesion just anterior to the ear with central umbilication and a 'rolled' edge. This is not a feature of naevi.*

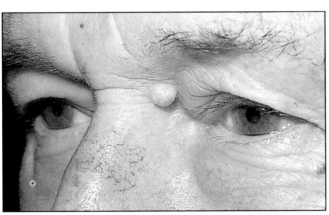

Figure 23.4 *Intradermal naevus: this site is common for BCC as well, but note that the lesion is skin-coloured and that there is a complete lack of surface telangiectasia.*

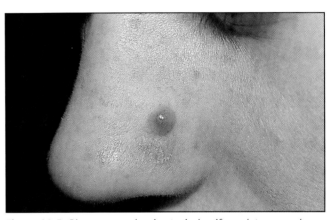

Figure 23.5 *Blue naevus, showing typical uniform slate-grey colour.*

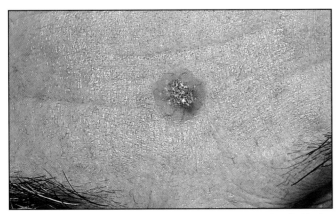

Figure 23.6 *Pigmented basal cell carcinoma: pigmentation is blacker and coarser than in naevi.*

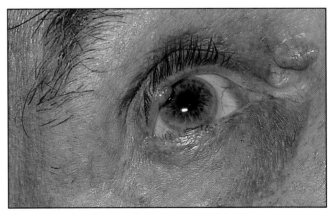

Figure 23.7 *Basal cell carcinoma of the medial canthus, and neurofibroma at the margin of the upper eyelid: this demonstrates how similar in appearance these two disorders can be.*

24 Basal cell carcinoma v. sebaceous hyperplasia

Common presenting feature: umbilicated facial papule.

Rationale for comparison: an incorrect diagnosis may lead to unnecessary surgery, as sebaceous hyperplasia is a benign condition.

Other differential diagnoses: other skin appendage neoplasia (e.g. trichofolliculomas, syringomas, hidrocystomas); molluscum contagiosum; seborrhoeic keratoses; nodular elastoidosis; senile comedones.

Conclusion and key points: sebaceous hyperplasia can usually be differentiated from basal cell carcinoma (BCC) by its yellowish colour and characteristic shape (it is always umbilicated with a depressed centre and rather cobblestoned periphery, even in small lesions), finite growth in size, and tendency for multiple lesions. Sebaceous hyperplasia has no pathological significance. A syndrome of sebaceous adenomas and carcinomas, which is associated with internal malignancy (Muir–Torre syndrome), is not likely to be confused with sebaceous hyperplasia; sebaceous adenomas are waxy, pink, or yellowish nodules, while sebaceous carcinoma may resemble BCC but has a predilection for the upper eyelid, which is a very rare site for BCC.

Comparative features		
Disorder	**Basal cell carcinoma (BCC)**	**Sebaceous hyperplasia**
Age	Middle-age onward, occasionally younger	
Sex	Either	
Family history	Non-specific	
Sites	Any part of face, including lower eyelid, nose, retroauricular	Mainly cheeks, forehead, temples
Symptoms	None	
Signs common to both	Smooth-surfaced facial papule	
Discriminatory signs	Small lesions are usually dome-shaped rather than umbilicated. Large lesions may ulcerate and crust. BCCs progressively increase in size. Typical BCCs have pearly grey colour, and surface telangiectasia; these features are most easily visualized if the skin is stretched.	Usually multiple. Yellowish colour. Close inspection demonstrates a 'doughnut' shape made up of several papules with an umbilicated centre.
Associated features	Solar damage is commonly associated with either	
Important tests	Histological confirmation and removal	None: no treatment required
Additional points	May also be confused with other appendage neoplasia including syringomas (multiple, flesh coloured, usually on lower eyelids), and trichoepitheliomas (usually around the nose; multiple or solitary lesions)	

Further reading:
p. 46, p. 86.

References

Miller SJ. Biology of basal cell carcinoma. *J Am Acad Dermatol* 1991; **24**:1–13, 161–75.

Schwarz RA, Torre DP. The Muir–Torre syndrome: a 25-year retrospect. *J Am Acad Dermatol* 1995; **33**:90–104.

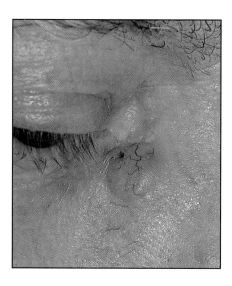

Figure 24.1 *Basal cell carcinoma of the medial canthus: this is also a common site for large comedones. Note the surface telangiectosia.*

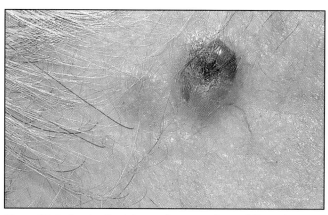

Figure 24.2 *Basal cell carcinoma demonstrating umbilicated centre in a larger lesion: the smaller adjacent yellowish-brown lesion is a seborrhoeic keratosis.*

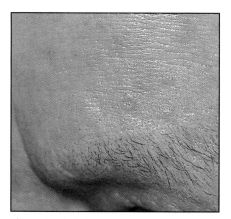

Figure 24.3 *Sebaceous hyperplasia: close-up view demonstrating yellowish colour, cobblestoned pattern of the border, and central umbilication, which would usually not be apparent in a basal cell carcinoma of this small size.*

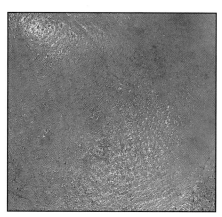

Figure 24.4 *Sebaceous hyperplasia: multiple lesions of similar morphology are reassuring.*

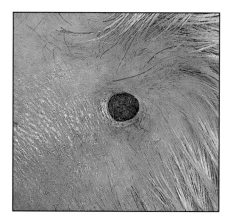

Figure 24.5 *Marsupialized epidermoid cysts: these are often confused with basal cell carcinoma and other skin malignancies. The contents may be expressed through the greatly dilated punctum.*

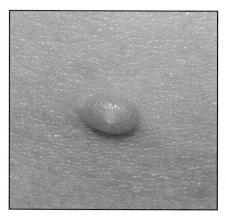

Figure 24.6 *Solitary molluscum in an adult: in this age-group, mollusca may be large and atypical compared with childhood (Fig. 65.3 p. 130).*

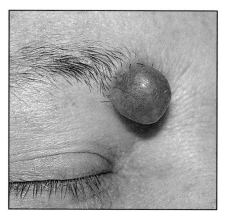

Figure 24.7 *Pilomatrixoma: this is a large nodular skin appendage neoplasm derived from hair root sheath.*

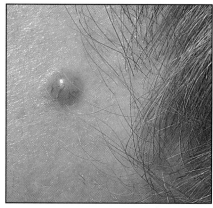

Figure 24.8 *Nodular basal cell carcinoma: this resembles a hidrocystoma or other skin appendage neoplasm—note similarity to Fig. 24.7.*

25 Cysts v. intradermal naevi

Common presenting feature: skin-coloured facial nodule(s).

Rationale for comparison: dome-shaped intradermal naevi are commonly mistaken for cysts. They are very common on the face and usually require no intervention. If they are treated surgically, the best cosmetic result is usually achieved by shave excision, whereas cysts require formal excision and cannot be treated by the simpler shave technique.

Other differential diagnoses: other types of naevus; skin appendage neoplasia; acne cysts; warts; molluscum contagiosum; neurofibromas; lipomas; fibroepithelial polyps ('skin tags').

Conclusion and key points: intradermal naevi are common on the face, but are often referred to dermatology clinics for diagnosis. They can usually be differentiated from cysts by virtue of having some degree of fine brown epidermal pigmentation, but some are skin-coloured as they have intradermal naevus cells only and are covered by normal epidermis. Naevi have a distinct edge which projects up from normal skin, whereas cysts are deeper and the skin stretched over them forms a shallow dome. Hairs are often present in naevi but not in cysts. The presence of a punctum is characteristic of epidermoid cysts but is not a feature of naevi, though it may not be visible in all cysts. Surgical techniques, if required, are different for the two disorders.

Comparative features		
Disorder	**Cyst**	**Intradermal naevus**
Age	Any, usually young adulthood	Mostly >30 yr
Sex	Either	
Family history	Non-specific	
Sites	Any, especially around ears	Any, especially cheeks, forehead
Symptoms	None unless secondary infection, which causes tenderness and swelling, with discharge of foul-smelling macerated keratin when punctured	None unless secondary folliculitis, which causes itch or tenderness, sometimes with erythema and/or swelling
Signs common to both	Dome-shaped skin-coloured nodule(s)	
Discriminatory signs	Epidermoid cysts are palpable as smooth firm subcutaneous nodules. Because the cyst is deep to the firm fibrous dermis, it produces a shallow dome-shaped protrusion. There may be a visible punctum. The overlying skin has normal colour and is mobile over the cyst (unless tethered due to previous rupture) but may appear stretched; the underlying cyst is firm and may be visibly white if the overlying skin is stretched.	There is often some degree of residual fine pigmentation. There may be prominent hairs or follicular orifices. Naevi have a sharper and steeper junction with adjacent skin compared with cysts. They have a rubbery texture, and the surface is a smooth dome-shaped or occasionally cobblestoned outline.
Associated features	May occur in acne	Often multiple
Important tests	None	
Treatment	Usually none. If excision is performed, the entire sac needs to be removed to prevent recurrence or inflammation.	None; shave excision is cosmetically neatest if treatment is required.

Further reading:
p. 12, p. 46, p. 160–164.

References
Green A, Siskind V, Green L. The incidence of melanocytic naevi in adolescent children in Queensland, Australia. *Melanoma Res* 1995; 5:155–60.

Hudson–Peacock MJ, Bishop J, Lawrence CM. Shave excision of benign papular naevocytic naevi. *Br J Plast Surg* 1995; 48:318–22.

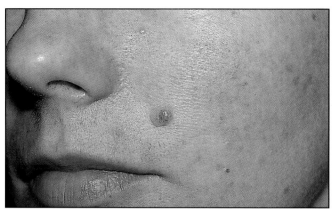

Figure 25.1 *Benign pigmented intradermal naevus on the lip: note the uniform colour and pigmentary pattern.*

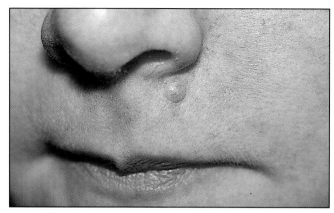

Figure 25.2 *Benign, non-pigmented, intradermal naevus on the cheek.*

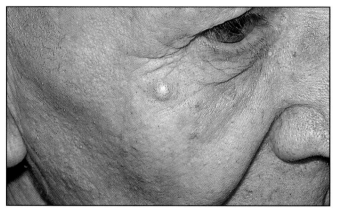

Figure 25.3 *Cyst on the cheek, demonstrating a whitish colour due to being visible through the skin which is stretched over it.*

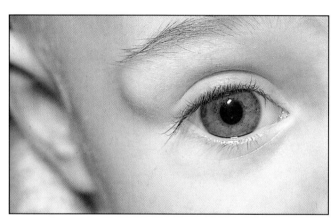

Figure 25.4 *True dermoid cyst: the eyebrow and temple region is a typical site. Note that this type of cyst is much rarer than the usual skin cysts that are correctly termed epidermoid cysts.*

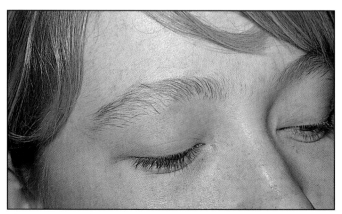

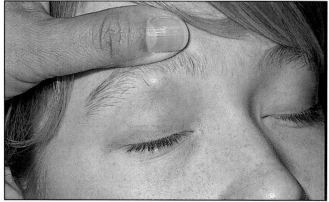

Figures 25.5 and 25.6 *Epidermoid cyst in the eyebrow: the lesion has been made more visible by stretching the overlying skin.*

26 Squamous cell carcinoma v. keratoacanthoma

Common presenting feature: an enlarging, keratinizing, nodule.

Rationale for comparison: these two disorders may be very difficult to differentiate, both clinically and pathologically, but have a very different prognosis. Keratoacanthomas (KAs) spontaneously regress, whereas squamous cell carcinoma (SCC) is potentially metastatic and may by fatal.

Other differential diagnoses: actinic keratosis (see p. 78); other causes of cutaneous horn (see Table); localized crusted lesions (e.g. basal cell carcinoma, dental sinus); rarer tumours (e.g. atypical fibroxanthoma, sebaceous epithelioma).

Conclusion and key points: it is vital to realize that even the combination of clinical and histological features may not provide a definite distinction between these disorders, in which case the lesion should be treated as SCC. In general, keratoacanthomas are faster growing than SCC, but stop growing after 2–3 months; they are typically symmetrical, have a formed central horn, and have a bolstered shoulder of skin stretched around the tumour. As they spontaneously involute, the horn may be lost, and a crateriform scar develops. A longer history of slow growth, asymmetrical shape, infiltrative edge, or presence of crust rather than a formed horn, should be assumed to indicate SCC.

Either of these may also occur on the chronically sun-exposed skin of the dorsal hands and forearms, but a definitive diagnosis of keratoacanthoma is more important on the face where skin surgery is technically more difficult.

Comparative features		
Disorder	**Squamous cell carcinoma (SCC)**	**Keratoacanthoma (KA)**
Age	Mostly >60 yr	Mostly >50 yr
Sex	Male predominance	
Family history	Non-specific	
Sites	Mainly sun-exposed skin of the face, but also hands, forearms, scalp, lower legs. On lips, tends to affect lower lip at vermilion border.	Sun-exposed skin, usually face, scalp, hands, or forearms. Upper lip lesions are more common than lower lip.
Symptoms	Often none, may be painful. History is of progressive increase in size, often at the site of a pre-existing smaller keratosis	None except history of rapid growth; the size should not increase beyond a 3-month period.
Signs common to both	Enlarging keratinizing nodule. Both may occur as multiple lesions in immunosuppressed patients; both are commonly associated with other signs of solar damage and actinic keratoses at other sites.	
Discriminatory signs	Usually a poorly demarcated or infiltrating edge, or surrounding flatter actinic keratosis. In SCC with rapid growth, the surface is usually crusted rather than having a formed horn.	A well formed horn (which may fall off in the involuting phase), yellowish bolstered skin edge, and a symmetrical shouldered central crater. No palpable changes occur beyond the lesion.
Associated features	The presence of lymphadenopathy almost certainly indicates SCC.	Occasionally multiple in rare inherited syndromes
Important tests	Excision of the SCC with histological assessment (or radiotherapy after incisional biopsy); clinical assessment of regional lymph nodes to determine the presence of metastatic disease.	Excision, curettage, or radiotherapy. Clinically typical lesions, especially those which present in the static or regressing phase, may be left to regress spontaneously but should be carefully observed to confirm involution.
Laboratory distinction	Confident distinction between SCC and KA may be impossible even after careful clinicopathological assessment. In such cases the tumour should be treated as an SCC, with appropriate follow-up.	

Further reading:
p. 46, p. 48, p. 54, p. 78, p. 128, p. 154, p. 156.

References

Dinehart SM, Pollack SV. Metastases from squamous cell carcinoma of skin and lip. *J Am Acad Dermatol* 1989; **21**:241–8.

Johnson TM, *et al*. Squamous cell carcinoma of the skin (excluding lip and oral mucosa). *J Am Acad Dermatol* 1992; **26**:467–84.

Schwartz RA. Keratoacanthoma. *J Am Acad Dermatol* 1994; **30**:1–19.

Cause of cutaneous horns	
Solar neoplasia	Actinic keratosis, SCC, keratoacanthoma
Infective	Viral warts
Benign epidermal neoplasia	Seborrhoeic keratosis, squamous papilloma, digitate keratoses

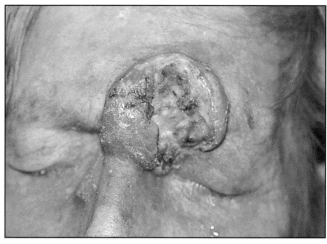

Figure 26.1 *Squamous cell carcinoma of upper eyelid: note asymmetry of ulceration and crusting.*

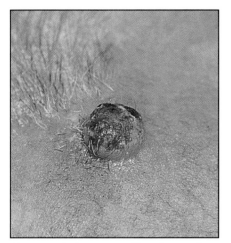

Figure 26.2 *Squamous cell carcinoma of cheek: note that this is crusted but has no formed horn.*

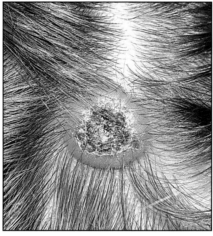

Figure 26.3 *Keratoacanthoma of scalp, with precise symmetry of the bolstered base.*

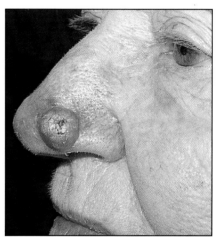

Figure 26.4 *Keratoacanthoma of nasal tip, a common site.*

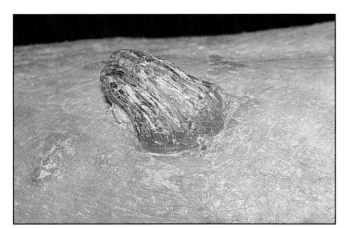

Figure 26.5 *Actinic keratosis: this is a large 'cutaneous horn' with a hypertrophic base but does not have the bolstered and rather yellowish colour of a keratoacanthoma. The horn also arises from the entire lesion rather than from a central crater. The clinical differential diagnosis is between a hypertrophic actinic keratosis and an early squamous cell carcinoma.*

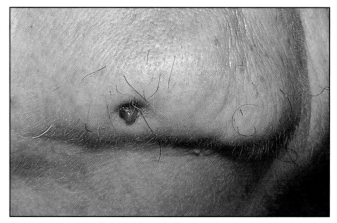

Figure 26.6 *Dental sinus: these lesions produce a variable central scab or crust, but do not have the basal hypertrophy of an epidermal neoplasm.*

27 Actinic keratosis of ear v. chondrodermatitis nodularis

Common presenting feature: nodule on rim of ear.

Rationale for comparison: chondrodermatitis may require treatment because of pain, which may be sufficient to disturb sleep. Actinic keratoses may often be left untreated if small, but do have some malignant potential. The most appropriate treatments for the two disorders are quite different.

Other differential diagnoses: squamous cell carcinoma; occasionally follicular keratoses or comedones; basal cell carcinoma (uncommon on edge of pinna); dermal lesions (e.g. keloid scar, granuloma annulare, gout).

Conclusion and key points: chondrodermatitis can usually be identified confidently because it is painful (marked tenderness on pressure, typically waking patients from sleep), has a specific site distribution on the ear (see figures), is usually on the ear that the individual sleeps on, and lacks the formed keratinization which is characteristic of actinic keratoses. Actinic keratoses, if they require treatment, are usually treated by cryotherapy; alternatives are topical 5-fluorouracil, curettage, or local excision. Treatment of chondrodermatitis is directed at the underlying cartilage inflammation rather than primarily at the skin. Some lesions of chondrodermatitis nodularis will respond to simply avoiding local pressure; some resolve after intralesional corticosteroid injection; but the best treatment is shave excision of the underlying cartilage.

Comparative features		
Disorder	**Chondrodermatitis nodularis**	**Actinic (solar) keratosis**
Age	Any; increases with age	Usually elderly
Sex	Either, but site on ear varies (mainly on helix in men, and antihelix in women)	Either, but actinic keratosis on the ears is more common in men than women
Family history	Non-specific	
Sites	The side of the helix or antihelix (other sites are rare unless due to direct injury, radiotherapy, frostbite etc). Usually affects the ear that patients lie on when asleep	Superior or posterior edge of ear. Position on helical rim is different to chondrodermatitis (see Figures 27.2–27.6 opposite)
Symptoms	Tenderness or sharp pain on pressure. Typically the pain wakes patients when they lie on the affected ear.	Usually none or minor discomfort, but larger lesions can be painful due to hard keratin. Lesions which are persistently painful even without being subjected to local pressure raise the suspicion of squamous cell carcinoma.
Signs common to both	Nodule on ear	
Discriminatory signs	Specific site. Pain is out of proportion to the visible lesion. May have an umbilicated centre, and may be crusted centrally but not keratinizing	Specific site. Diffuse surface keratinization
Associated features	None. Actinic damage elsewhere is not uncommon as patients are often elderly.	Actinic damage elsewhere is expected.
Important tests	None. If excision is necessary, shave removal of the underlying cartilage to leave smooth edges is the treatment of choice.	If lesions are painful, consider secondary infection (in which case send a swab for bacteriology) or development of squamous cell carcinoma (in which case excise the lesion). Induration which is not caused by simple keratinization suggests squamous cell carcinoma.

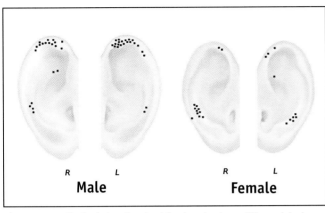

Figure 27.1 *Typical sites involved in chondrodermatitis nodularis (redrawn with permission from Lawrence CM., op. cit.).*

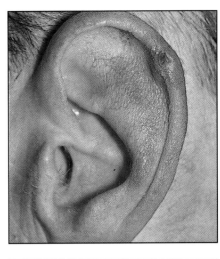

Figure 27.2 *Chondrodermatitis nodularis: shown at typical site on the helix of the ear.*

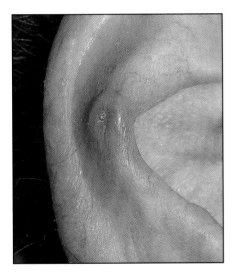

Figure 27.3 *Chondrodermatitis nodularis: shown on the antihelix. Central umbilication is common but note lack of keratinization.*

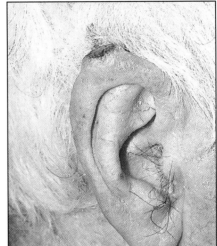

Figure 27.4 *Squamous cell carcinoma affecting the upper part of the rim of the ear. Note the thickened base.*

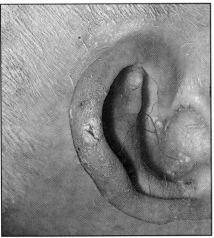

Figure 27.5 *Actinic keratosis affecting the ear, showing diffuse keratinization (and numerous smaller keratoses of the ear and scalp) (see also Fig. 20.6).*

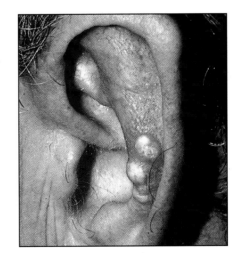

Figure 27.6 *Gout: the tophi on the ear are white-coloured deposits which are within the tissues, and therefore have a smooth surface.*

Further reading:
p. 40, p. 78, p. 154.

References
Drake LA, *et al*. Guidelines of care for actinic keratoses. *J Am Acad Dermatol* 1995; **32**:95–8.
Frost CA, Green AC. Epidemiology of solar keratoses. *Br J Dermatol* 1994; **131**:455–64.

Hudson–Peacock MJ, Cox NH, Lawrence CM. Long-term effectiveness of cartilage removal for the treatment of chondrodermatitis nodularis. *Br J Dermatol* 1995; **133**(Suppl 45):46.
Lawrence CM. The treatment of chondrodermatitis nodularis with cartilage removal alone. *Arch Dermatol* 1991; **127**:530–5.

28 Flat seborrhoeic keratosis v. solar lentigo

Common presenting feature: flat brown macule, usually multiple, at sun-exposed sites.

Rationale for comparison: these two disorders are often confused. The term 'liver spots' is often applied to either diagnosis.

Other differential diagnoses: lentigo maligna; pigmented actinic keratosis, (p. 40); discoid lupus erythematosus, Fig. 15.5.

Conclusion and key points: seborrhoeic keratoses on the face may be virtually flat unlike the thicker keratotic or waxy lesions which are more typical on the trunk. The surface is, however, rough or warty in texture on close examination. A solar lentigo has a more uniform brown colour and finer surface scale. Distinction can be very difficult, and is usually not of great importance provided the benign nature of both diagnoses is recognized.

Comparative features		
Disorder	**Flat seborrhoeic keratoses**	**Solar lentigo**
Age	Mostly >60 yr	Mostly >40 yr
Sex	Either	
Family history	Non-specific	
Sites	Any site. They are usually more warty on the trunk, but flat lesions on the legs are not uncommon and also cause diagnostic problems (see Fig. 78.8).	Any sun-exposed site (most commonly face, forearms, hands)
Symptoms	None	
Signs common to both	Virtually flat, mid-brown, slightly scaly plaque	
Discriminatory signs	Seborrhoeic keratoses have a more keratotic surface, in which small white dots formed by 'pearls' of keratin may be visible. The margin is usually fairly sharply defined. Some degree of colour variation or speckling is common.	These have a uniform colour, a slightly scaly rather than a rough surface, and often a relatively poorly defined margin.
Associated features	Often multiple	Solar damage
Important tests	None	

Further reading:
p. 40, p. 78, p. 160, p. 162.

References
Cohen LM. Lentigo maligna and lentigo maligna melanoma. *J Am Acad Dermatol* 1995; **33**:923–36.

Sanderson KV. The structure of seborrhoeic keratoses. *Br J Dermatol* 1968; **80**:588–93.
Yeatman JM, Kilkenny M, Marks R. The prevalence of seborrhoeic keratoses in an Australian population: does sunlight play a part in their frequency? *Br J Dermatol* 1997; **137**:411–414.

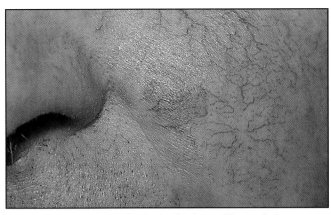

Figure 28.1 *Lentigo on the cheek: this is a uniform pale brown, smooth, flat lesion.*

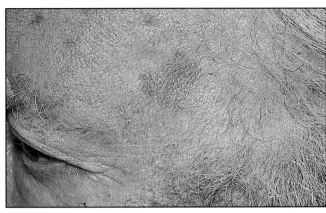

Figure 28.2 *Lentigo on the temple, same patient as in Fig. 28.1.*

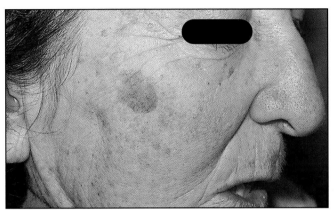

Figure 28.3 *Seborrhoeic keratosis on the cheek: slight colour variation or speckling is common in these lesions.*

Figure 28.4 *Seborrhoeic keratosis: very thin lesions may have a rather pinker colour but, typically, very sharply demarcated border.*

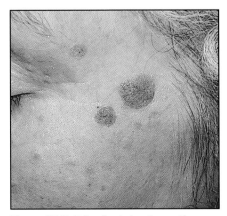

Figure 28.5 *Seborrhoeic keratoses: these are more typical thickened, greasy, muddy-brown lesions.*

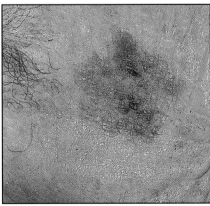

Figure 28.6 *Seborrhoeic keratosis on the temple: this demonstrates a greater degree of colour variation.*

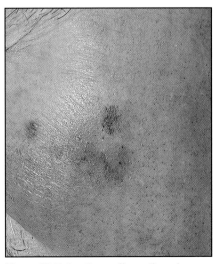

Figure 28.7 *Lentigo maligna: the colour change includes black speckling and some areas of pigment loss.*

Common presenting feature: erythema, scaling, and fissuring of the palms and/or soles.

Rationale for comparison: these two disorders may be very difficult to differentiate but the importance of a firm diagnosis is the much wider range of therapeutic options for psoriasis.

Other differential diagnoses: specific forms of dermatitis (contact dermatitis, hyperkeratotic dermatitis of palms and soles, lichen simplex of palms or insteps); fungal infection; pityriasis rubra pilaris; keratodermas (p.60);

palmoplantar pustulosis (p. 66).

Conclusion and key points: these two disorders can be difficult to differentiate clinically, and unfortunately in such cases, histological examination does not usually resolve the issue. The coexistence of specific nail changes may be helpful (p. 174), and there may be lesions at other sites. Lesions of psoriasis tend to be more sharply demarcated. It is always prudent to send skin scrapings for mycology to exclude fungal infection (p. 62) because of the difficulty in differentiating this disorder from dermatitis or psoriasis on hands and/or feet.

Comparative features

Disorder	Chronic psoriasis	Chronic dermatitis
Age	Adult, any (onset of psoriasis has peaks in early adult years and sixth or seventh decade, but this is not a useful discriminator for patients with involvement of palms and/or soles in isolation)	Adult, any
Sex	Either	Mainly males
Family history	May be positive	May be atopic
Sites	Palms and/or soles. May be lesions at other body sites	Palms and/or soles
Symptoms	None, itch, soreness if fissured	Itch is a more prominent symptom in dermatitis than in psoriasis. Fissured lesions are sore in either disorder.
Signs common to both	Chronic erythema, scaling, fissuring	
Discriminatory signs	By comparison with dermatitis, affected areas have sharper demarcation from normal skin, and scales are larger and more silvery in colour. Linear (sometimes grooved or umbilicated) bands of hyperkeratosis (Caro-Senear ridges), Fig. 29.5, at the sides of fingers or borders of the palms are uncommon but diagnostic of psoriasis.	Involved areas are less well demarcated, and with less well formed scale. fissuring is more common than in psoriasis, and there may be episodic more acute changes with vesicles (see p. 66). Chronic paronychia is common in dermatitis.
Associated features	Nail changes of psoriasis (p. 174), psoriasis elsewhere (commonest sites are elbows, knees, scalp, gluteal)	Nail changes in dermatitis (p. 174) are less specific than in psoriasis, and dermatitis at other sites is not frequent except in atopic individuals.
Important tests	Biopsy is occasionally helpful but may be painful on palms and soles, and results are often not specific.	Patch testing may be required.

Further reading:
p. 2, p. 42, pp. 60–68, pp. 80–84, p. 102, p. 110, p. 118, p. 120, p. 174, p. 176.

References

Caro MR, Senear FE. Psoriasis of the hands: non-pustular type. *Arch Dermatol Syphilol* 1947; **56**:629–32.
Larko O. Problem sites: scalp, palm and sole, and nail. *Dermatol Clinics* 1995; **13**:771–7.
Samitz MH, Albom JJ. Palmar psoriasis. *Arch Dermatol Syphilol* 1951; **64**:199–204.

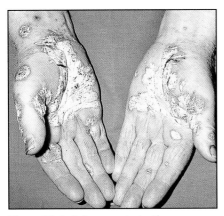

Figure 29.1 *Palmar psoriasis: there are typical discrete silvery hyperkeratotic plaques.*

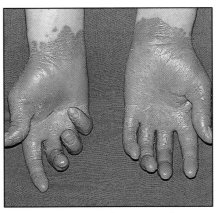

Figure 29.2 *More erythematous palmar psoriasis: a sharp cut-off as shown here favours psoriasis rather than dermatitis, and the beefy erythema is unlikely in a dermatitis.*

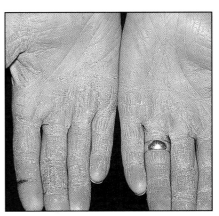

Figure 29.3 *Chronic palmar dermatitis: there is diffuse scaling with fissuring at flexures.*

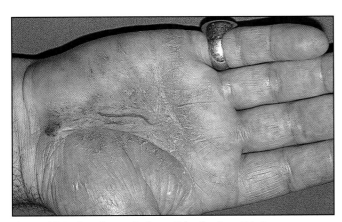

Figure 29.4 *Hyperkeratotic dermatitis of palms: this is a therapeutically difficult frictional disorder, which can be difficult to differentiate from psoriasis.*

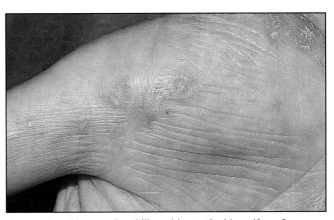

Figure 29.5 *Linear and umbilicated keratotic ridges (Caro–Senear ridges): these are diagnostic of psoriasis.*

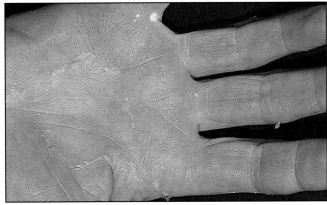

Figure 29.6 *Palmar peeling: this may occur as a variant of palmar dermatitis. It can also occur as a seasonal disorder or after systemic infections.*

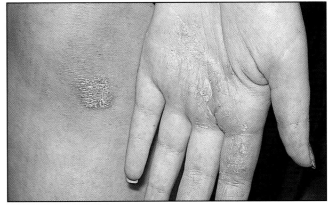

Figure 29.7 *The diagnosis of this chronic palmar eruption in a child was either dermatitis or psoriasis, but remained uncertain for 5 years, at which stage she developed psoriasis on one knee, as shown.*

Common presenting feature: diffuse hyperkeratosis of palms and/or soles.

Rationale for comparison: diagnostic confusion is unlikely except in young patients; therapeutic differences are important.

Other differential diagnoses: other keratodermas, e.g. simple callosities; keratoderma climactericum; pitted keratolysis (p. 68); chronic dermatitis (p. 58, Fig. 31.3); fungal infection; pityriasis rubra pilaris.

Conclusion and key points: diffuse palmoplantar keratoderma causes few symptoms and is therefore unlikely to be confused with dermatitis, but may be confused with psoriasis. It produces a uniform, yellowish-coloured, diffuse thickening of keratin rather than the whiter scaling that occurs in psoriasis, and has a sharp cut-off at the border of the palm and sole. There is often an erythematous border around the hyperkeratotic skin, and the same process may affect the dorsal distal phalanx and knuckles.

Comparative features		
Disorder	**Chronic psoriasis**	**Diffuse palmoplantar keratoderma (tylosis)**
Age	Diagnostic confusion is most likely if onset is in childhood, but this is relatively uncommon	Usually apparent by age 4
Sex	Either	
Family history	May be positive	Autosomal dominant inheritance
Sites	Palms and/or soles, may also be present at other body sites	Diffuse palm and sole involvement that may extend to dorsum (knuckles, distal fingers and toes)
Symptoms	None, itch, discomfort if fissured	Reduced mobility of hand, no itch but may fissure. There may be a smell from macerated thickened keratin.
Signs common to both	Palm and/or sole hyperkeratosis	
Discriminatory signs	Diffuse erythema as well as scaling, often variable and spared areas	Complete involvement of both palms and both soles. The hyperkeratosis appears yellowish and waxy rather than the looser scale that occurs in psoriasis. There is a sharp border, with a rim of erythema, at the margin of palms and soles.
Associated features	Nail changes or psoriasis elsewhere may be apparent	Similar changes may occur over knuckles, elbows, or knees. There is an association with carcinoma of oesophagus in some kindreds, but no associated features in the majority of patients.
Important tests	None	Investigate for oesophageal carcinoma in the very rare individuals from an affected kindred. Skin biopsy and electron microscopy may be important to distinguish between tylosis, epidermolytic hyperkeratosis, and other types of palmoplantar keratoderma in order to offer genetic counselling and to help predict treatment response.

Further reading:
p. 58, p. 62, p. 64, p. 68, p. 82, p. 84, p. 110, p. 118, p. 120, p. 174, p. 176.

References
Cohen PR, Prystowsky JH. Pityriasis rubra pilaris: a review of diagnosis and treatment. *J Am Acad Dermatol* 1989; **20**:801–7.
Farber EM, Nall L. Non-pustular palmoplantar psoriasis. *Cutis* 1992; **50**: 407–10.
Griffiths WAD. Pityriasis rubra pilaris. *Clin Exp Dermatol* 1980; **5**:105–12.

Marger RS, Marger D. Carcinoma of the esophagus and tylosis: a lethal genetic combination. *Cancer* 1993; **72**:17–19.
Marghescu S. Palmoplantar reactions. *Dermatology* 1994; **189**(Suppl 2):30–4.
Stevens HP, *et al.* Linkage of an American pedigree with palmoplantar kertoderma and malignancy (palmoplantar ectodermal dysplasia type III) to 17q24. *Arch Dermatol* 1996; **132**:640–51.

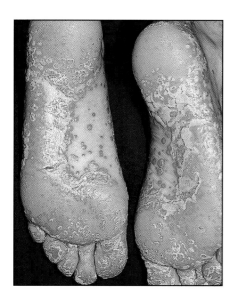

Figure 30.1
Acute exacerbation of chronic plantar psoriasis: note the loose scale and the scattered peripheral lesions on the insteps.

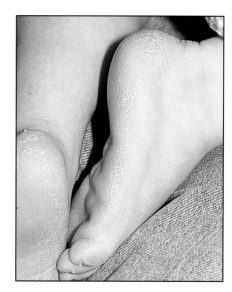

Figure 30.2
Diffuse keratoderma: note the yellowish waxy colour, erythematous proximal border, and sharp demarcation.

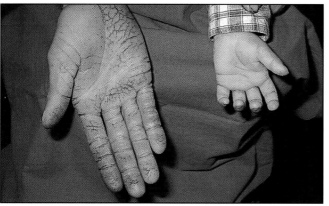

Figure 30.3 *Autosomal-dominant, diffuse, palmoplantar keratoderma in a father and son: relative sparing of creases is common, as is the more verrucous surface in adults.*

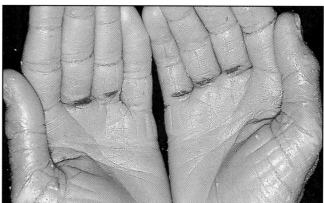

Figure 30.4 *Pityriasis rubra pilaris: palms and soles typically have a rather orange colour, with follicular lesions at other body sites (see also Fig.31.6 and 40.3). The purple colour in the fissures is an antiseptic paint.*

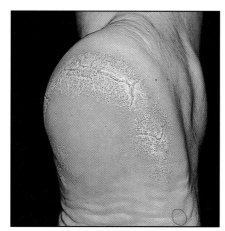

Figure 30.5 *Keratoderma climactericum: this is a symmetrical pattern of keratoderma which affects the border of the heels and other parts of the foot, typically seen in women in their sixth decade.*

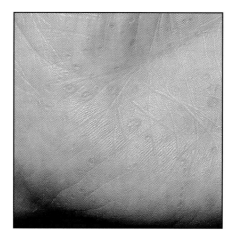

Figure 30.6 *Punctate keratoderma: this demonstrates the umbilicated appearance of the discrete palmar lesions. These lesions may be confused with Caro–Senear ridges of psoriasis (Fig. 29.5) but affect the central palm and sole rather than the border of the hands.*

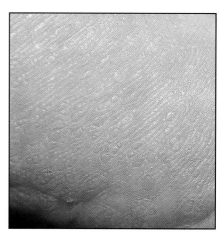

Figure 30.7 *Darier's disease: papular lesions on the palms are generally smaller and less keratinized than in punctate palmoplantar keratoderma.*

31 Chronic dermatitis v. fungal infection

Common presenting feature: chronic erythematous scaly palm and/or sole rash.

Rationale for comparison: these disorders are commonly confused but distinction is important as their treatment is fundamentally different, and is usually curative for fungal infection.

Other differential diagnoses: psoriasis (p. 58); pitted keratolysis of feet (p. 68); keratodermas (p. 60); pityriasis rubra pilaris, Fig. 30.4; chronic scabies of hands.

Conclusion and key points: confusion usually arises when there is a diffuse palm or sole rash. Fungal infection is usually less itchy than dermatitis. Most chronic palmar

fungal infection is caused by *Trichophyton rubrum*, which produces background erythema with fine white scaling predominantly in skin creases. A useful clue on the palms is that fungal infection is almost always asymmetrical and typically occurs with bilateral disease of the feet (one hand–two foot syndrome). By contrast, dermatitis of the hands usually affects both hands. Asymmetrical dermatitis (e.g. affecting the non-dominant hand in hairdressers and cooks, Figs. 31.4 and 38.6), is not associated with plantar disease. Always specifically examine the feet as patients may be unaware of diffuse fine scaling or toeweb disease, and always take mycology samples. Fungal disease of toenails is very commonly present in patients with diffuse plantar fungal infection, and the appearances may be similar to those of psoriasis.

Comparative features		
Disorder	**Chronic dermatitis**	**Fungal infection**
Age	Adult	
Sex	Either	Male predominance
Family history	Non-specific	
Sites	Palms and/or soles	Usually soles of feet, or one hand with both soles (one hand–two foot syndrome), typically including lateral toewebs and sometimes nails (especially feet)
Symptoms	Itch, pain if fissured	None, itch, hyperhidrosis, smelly feet
Signs common to both	Chronic erythematous scaling rash diffusely involving palmar or plantar surface; nail dystrophy	
Discriminatory signs	Presence of an acute vesicular component is more common in dermatitis but can occur in acute fungal infection (usually due to *Trichophyton mentagrophytes*). Toewebs are usually spared, but dermatitis may affect fingerwebs and dorsal surface of hands. Eczematous nail changes may be present.	Asymmetry is characteristic on hands but less frequent on feet. Palm involvement is almost always accompanied by involvement of soles but not the converse. Typically affects toewebs as well as more diffuse scaling; toenail involvement is common. Scale is fine and accentuated in crease lines.
Associated features	There may be dermatitis at other sites. Chronic paronychia is a feature of dermatitis rather than of dermatophyte fungal infection.	May be more typical annular fungal lesions at other sites. In more acute examples, a secondary eczematous 'id' eruption may occur at other body sites.
Important tests	Patch tests to exclude allergy (e.g. to footwear). Always send scale for mycology.	Send skin scrapings for mycology (Fig. 55.6) to confirm the infection prior to therapy, as palm/sole infections usually need systemic treatment.

Further reading:
p. 58, p. 60, p. 64–68, p. 76, p. 96, p. 102, p. 110, p. 118, p. 120, p. 170–176.

References
See p. 76.

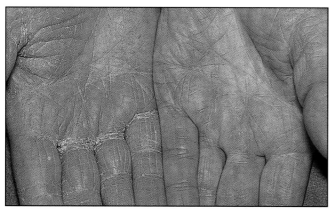

Figure 31.1 *Chronic palmar infection with* Trichophyton rubrum: *note asymmetrical distribution (typically unilateral, as in this case, but usually with bilateral plantar infection).*

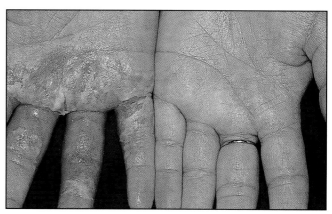

Figure 31.2 *Acute fungal infection of the hand: again, note typical asymmetry.*

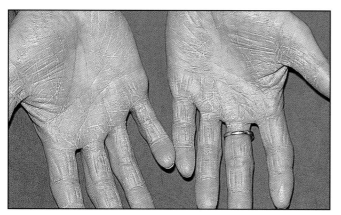

Figure 31.3 *Chronic dermatitis of the hands in a cook.*

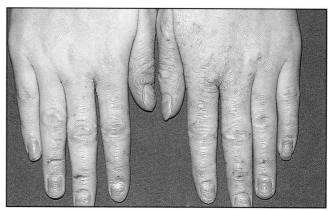

Figure 31.4 *Asymmetrical chronic dermatitis may cause diagnostic confusion. It is a common pattern in hairdressers (as in this case) because wet hair (+/− dyes, bleach, perm agents etc.) is mainly held between the fingers of the non-dominant hand.*

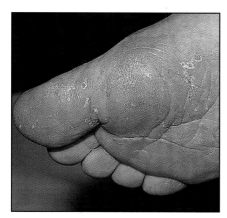

Figure 31.5 *Trichophyton rubrum infection on the sole: fungal infection of nails should be sought and treated to prevent recurrence of plantar infection.*

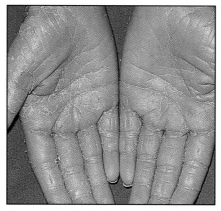

Figure 31.6 *Pityriasis rubra pilaris: this may be confused with dermatitis or tinea of palms. It is a symmetrical disorder with somewhat orange-coloured hyperkeratosis rather than the finer scaling of a dermatitis.*

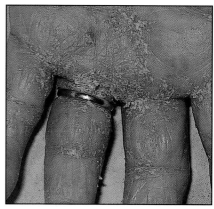

Figure 31.7 *Chronic scabies infestation is an important differential diagnosis of diffuse palmar scaling and crusting, and is usually most marked in the web spaces.*

Chronic dermatitis v. juvenile plantar dermatosis

Common presenting feature: plantar erythematous scaling eruption.

Rationale for comparison: Juvenile plantar dermatosis (JPD) is a childhood eruption which usually regresses spontaneously at or before puberty. It responds poorly to topical corticosteroids. Correct diagnosis is therefore important for prognosis and treatment.

Other differential diagnoses: tinea pedis; psoriasis.

Conclusion and key points: JPD is typically a symmetrical eruption in the 1–15 years age group (most cases occur at about 6 years of age). On the feet, it is limited to the weight-bearing plantar skin including pulps of toes, but occasionally it also affects the palms. JPD causes a characteristic glazed shiny redness, sometimes with fissuring, but not with a typical dermatitis scaling pattern. Chronic dermatitis of the soles in this age group is otherwise usually associated with overt atopic dermatitis at other sites, but can occasionally be caused by contact allergy to footwear. Extensive symmetrical tinea pedis (p. 62 and Fig. 34.4) is uncommon in children but may occur if masked by incorrect topical steroid therapy (tinea incognito, Figs. 55.1–55.5).

Comparative features		
Disorder	**Chronic dermatitis**	**Juvenile plantar dermatitis (JPD)**
Age	Uncommon in childhood	5–15 yr
Sex	Either	
Family history	Chronic palm or sole dermatitis in children usually occurs because of atopy, so most patients will have a family history of dermatitis or other atopic diseases.	Non-specific
Sites	Usually affects the dorsal as well as the plantar aspect of the foot in atopic dermatitis. Contact allergy may affect the sole and/or dorsum of the foot.	Weight-bearing area of sole including pulps of toes
Symptoms	Itch; discomfort and difficulty walking due to fissuring	None or some itch; discomfort and difficulty walking due to fissuring
Signs common to both	Erythema; fissuring of sole of foot	
Discriminatory signs	Extension onto dorsum of foot, eczematous nail changes. There may be features of atopic dermatitis elsewhere (note that the prevalence of JPD may be increased in atopics).	Glazed erythema rather than significant dry scaling, sharply localized to plantar skin, spares toewebs and does not extend onto the dorsum of the foot
Associated features	Atopic dermatitis, occasionally contact allergic or dermatitis, at other sites	Occasionally involves thenar/hypothenar areas of palm
Important tests	Patch tests are sometimes indicated if contact allergy is suspected.	
Treatment	Emollients, topical corticosteroids, antibiotics or antiseptics if fissured or weeping; bandaging	Avoid excessive stimulus of sweating by attention to footwear. Emollients. Topical corticosteroids for itch but not routinely. Reduce physical activity if symptoms are severe.

Further reading:
pp. 58–62, p. 68, p. 76, p. 110, p. 132.

References

Jepson LV. Dermatitis plantaris sicca; a retrospective study of children with recurrent dermatitis of the feet. *Acta Dermatovenereol* (Stockh) 1979; **59**:257.

Jones SK, English JSC, Forsyth A, *et al.* Juvenile plantar dermatosis: an 8-year follow up of 102 patients. *Clin Exp Dermatol* 1987; **12**:5–7.

McBride A, Cohen BA. Tinea pedis in children. *Am J Dis Child* 1992; **146**:844–7.

Verbov JL. Atopic dermatitis and the forefoot. *BMJ* 1978; **ii**:962.

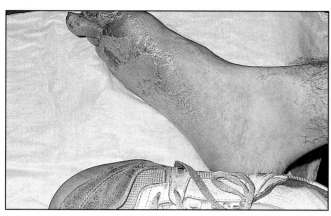

Figure 32.1 *Foot dermatitis in a young man caused by thiuram (a rubber chemical) in his shoes.*

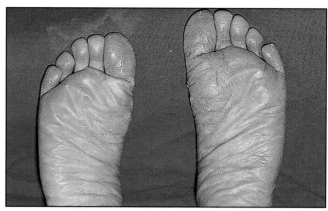

Figure 32.2 *Juvenile plantar dermatosis: there is symmetrical glazed shiny skin of the weight-bearing area of the soles, with a typical collodion-like appearance.*

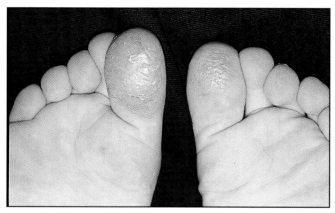

Figure 32.3 *Juvenile plantar dermatosis: involvement may be confined to pulps of toes.*

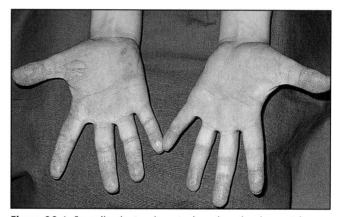

Figure 32.4 *Juvenile plantar dermatosis: palmar involvement is uncommon, but may occur in patients with severe plantar involvement.*

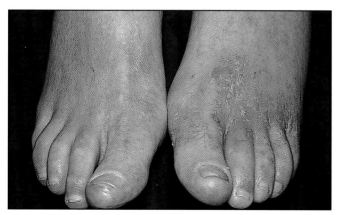

Figure 32.5 *Tinea pedis: this disorder may mimic juvenile plantar dermatosis but the latter does not extend onto the dorsum of the foot as shown here.*

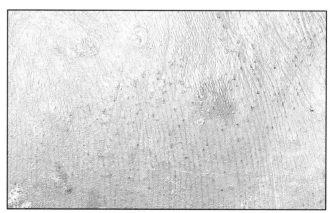

Figure 32.6 *Pompholyx vesicles: typically occur in dermatitis, but are not a common feature of juvenile plantar dermatosis (see also Fig. 33.3).*

33 Palmoplantar pustulosis v. pompholyx eczema

Common presenting feature: acute vesico-pustular eruption of hands or feet, especially palms or soles.

Rationale for comparison: different topical and systemic therapeutic options. Diagnostic difficulty arises because secondary infection of pompholyx may cause pustules, while vesicular lesions occur in early stages of palmaplantar pustulosis pustule formation.

Other differential diagnoses: scabies; fungal infection (especially *Trichophyton mentagrophytes*); secondary infection of other palm and/or sole eruptions; bullous pemphigoid; acropustulosis of infancy; pustular bacterid.

Conclusion and key points: palmoplantar pustulosis (PPP) is characterized by pustular lesions, usually about 5 mm in diameter, with various stages of lesion found simultaneously; early yellow pustules become green, then brown as they dry up and crust. The pustules occur on an erythematous background, with hyperkeratosis, scaling, and fissuring. PPP particularly affects the border of the heel, but may affect other parts of the hands or feet, including the periungual and subungual area. PPP is usually symmetrical when established, but is often initially asymmetrical in which case fungal infection must be excluded by taking samples for mycology. An interesting feature is the close association with cigarette smoking (90% of patients are, or were, smokers, at the onset of PPP). Pompholyx typically consists of tiny vesicles with larger, but still obviously multilocular, blisters in acute phases.

Comparative features		
Disorder	**Palmoplantar pustulosis (PPP)**	**Pompholyx eczema**
Age	Onset in middle-age	Any, especially young adult
Sex	Female predominance	Either
Family history	May be positive for psoriasis	Non-specific
Sites	Mainly affects the heel but may occur at any site on palm and/or sole. Nailbed pustules occur in up to 30% of patients, and lesions may occur on the dorsum of distal digits.	May be diffuse palm or sole involvement; when milder, typically affects sides of fingers
Symptoms	Tender in acute phase	Itch
Signs common to both	Vesicopustules of palms or soles	
Discriminatory signs	Pustules arise on an erythematous scaly so-called psoriasiform background. Most pustules are large, and pustules of different stages of evolution are typically present concurrently producing a polymorphic picture with yellow, green, and brown pustules (see figures). Nailbed pustules are a useful discriminatory feature when they are present.	There is a predominance of small vesicles, and particularly multilocular blisters. Commonly affects sides of fingers. If pustules are present, they generally represent secondary infection and are relatively monomorphic.
Associated features	Up to 30% of patients have psoriasis at other sites, but PPP has numerous clinical and laboratory differences from psoriasis. About 90% of patients are cigarette smokers at the onset of PPP, although stopping smoking does not cause remission. Monoarthritis and sternoclavicular or manubriosternal arthritis occur in 5–10% of cases.	
Important tests	Exclude fungal infection. Bacteriology swab if acute exacerbation	Patch test; bacteriology swabs if pustules

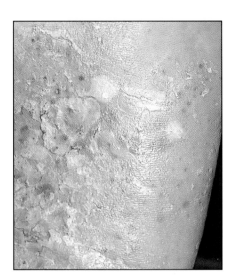

Figure 33.1
Palmoplantar pustolosis demonstrating typical large pustules in various stages of evolution.

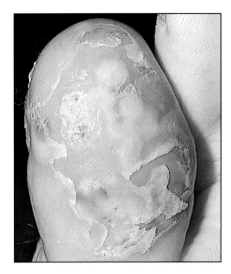

Figure 33.2
Palmoplantar pustolosis: close-up view of the same patient as in Fig. 33.1.

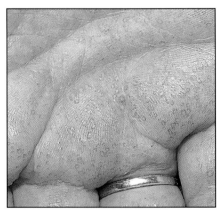

Figure 33.3
Pompholyx of the hand (see also Fig. 32.6) demonstrating tiny vesicles.

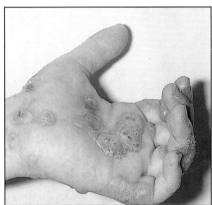

Figure 33.4
Pompholyx: this is a more acute example with large multilocular blisters.

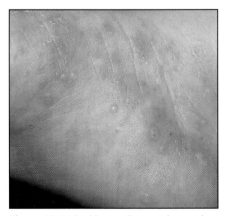

Figure 33.5 *Scabies: vesicopustules on the foot of a baby. This is a common site for scabies in this age-group.*

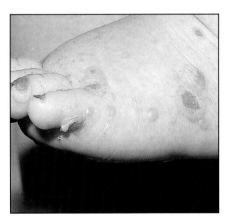

Figure 33.6 *Scabies in a baby: larger blisters may occur as shown here.*

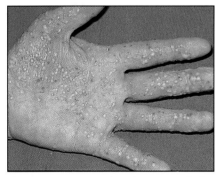

Figure 33.7 *Acute palmoplantar pustulosis, as an 'id' eruption in a patient with an acute contact dermatitis of the scalp. Note the scattered and monomorphic discrete pustules (compare with distribution of lesions in palmar plantar pustolosis, Fig. 33.1).*

Further reading:
pp. 58–64, p. 68, p. 106, p. 108, p. 114, p. 144.

References
Andrews GC, Machacek GF. Pustular bacterids of the hands and feet. *Arch Dermatol Syphilol* 1935; **32**:837–17.
Cox NH, Ray S. Neutrophil leukocyte morphology, cigarette smoking, and palmoplantar pustulosis. *Int J Dermatol* 1987; **26**:445–7.
O'Doherty CJ, MacIntyre C. Palmoplantar pustulosis and smoking. *BMJ* 1985; **291**:861–4.

Prendiville JS. Infantile acropustulosis—how often is it a sequel of scabies? *Pediatr Dermatol* 1995; **12**:275–6.
Thomsen K, Osterbye P. Pustulosis palmaris et plantaris. *Br J Dermatol* 1973; **89**: 293–6.
Vehara M. Pustulosis palmaris et plantaris, evolutionary sequence from vesicular to pustular lesions. *Semin Dermatol* 1983; **2**:51–6.

34 Pitted keratolysis v. tinea pedis

Common presenting features: smelly feet, scaling rash on soles of feet.

Rationale for comparison: these two disorders are often confused diagnostically but have a different aetiology and hence different treatments.

Other differential diagnoses: dermatitis; psoriasis; juvenile plantar dermatosis; soft corn in toewebs.

Conclusion and key points: pitted keratolysis is a corynebacterial infection which occurs in sweaty feet. It is characterized by smelly, yellowish, macerated keratin. There is usually focal peeling and pitting, and lesions are often annular and sharply demarcated. The pulps of the toes are often affected when pitted keratolysis involves the forefoot. Tinea pedis may present with areas of macerated skin but is particularly prominent in the toeclefts. Tinea spreading onto the plantar skin usually causes erythema with fine scaling, but may cause blistering and weeping. Fungal infections may also spread to the dorsum of the foot, whereas pitted keratolysis does not occur at this site.

Comparative features		
Disorder	**Pitted keratolysis**	**Tinea pedis**
Age	Mainly teens, young adult onset, but may occur in older age groups	
Sex	Male predominance	
Family history	Non-specific	
Sites	Sole of foot, usually forefoot where pulp of toes is often affected. Usually symmetrical	Toewebs, usually 4th/5th cleft but may be 3rd/4th also; may extend onto sole or dorsum of the foot
Symptoms	None, smell	Itch
Signs common to both	Macerated scaling of sole of foot	
Discriminatory signs	Yellowish colour on sole, focal peeling and pitting, annular shapes, usually both feet	Lateral toecleft sites; erythema and loose scaling if affects adjacent sole or dorsum of foot. Often asymmetrical in earliest stages
Associated features	Sweaty feet	There may be associated fungal nail dystrophy.
Important tests	None routinely required; soaking foot in water for 15 minutes will accentuate the keratolytic appearance.	Mycology samples, particularly if systemic therapy is considered
Treatment	This is a corynebacterial infection which responds to topical antibiotics such as fusidic acid or mupirocin; measures to reduce sweating (topical antiperspirants, attention to footwear) also help.	Fungal infections may respond to topical or oral agents (depending on severity) including imidazoles, triazoles, allylamines.

Further reading:
pp. 58–66, p. 76, p. 110, p. 170–176.

References
Day RD, Harkless LB, Reyzelman AM. Evaluation and management of the interdigital corn: a literature review. *Clin Pod Med & Surg* 1996; **13(2)**:201–6.
Lamberg SI. Symptomatic pitted keratolysis. *Arch Dermatol* 1969; **100**:10–11.
Zaias N. Pitted and ringed keratolysis. *J Am Acad Dermatol* 1982; **7**:787–91.

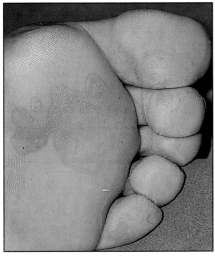

Figure 34.1 *Pitted keratolysis showing a well-demarcated yellowish annular lesion and involvement of pulps of toes.*

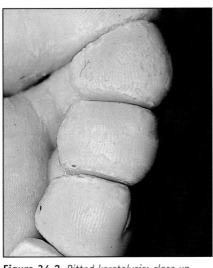

Figure 34.2 *Pitted keratolysis: close-up view of a patient with lesions affecting pulps of toes.*

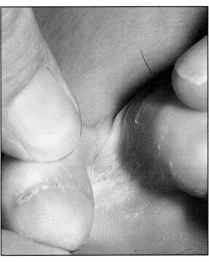

Figure 34.3 *Toeweb tinea pedis.*

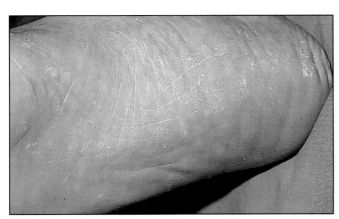

Figure 34.4 *Tinea pedis due to* Trichophyton rubrum, *showing a typical erythema and fine scaling.*

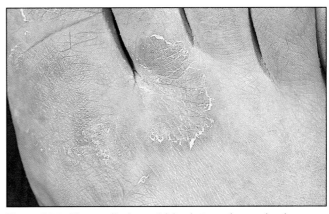

Figure 34.5 *Tinea pedis due to* Trichophyton rubrum, *showing extension onto dorsum of foot.*

Figure 34.6 *Soft corn under toe.*

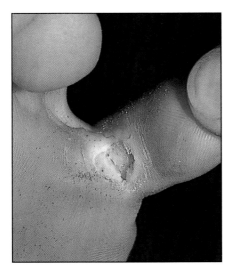

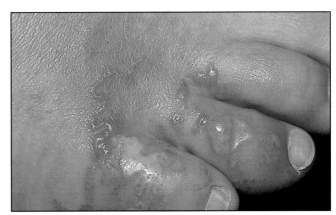

Figure 34.7 *Cutaneous larva migrans (dog hookworm infestation): this may give rise to diagnostic confusion when it occurs around toes, as it may cause annular patterns and blistering.*

69

35 Plantar wart (verruca) v. corn

Common presenting feature: painful keratotic lesions on the weight-bearing area of the sole of the foot.

Rationale for comparison: these disorders may be confused diagnostically, but therapy is different; corns require avoidance of localized pressure.

Other differential diagnoses: other localized callosities; eccrine poroma; talon noir of heel; punctate keratoderma (see Fig. 30.6); carcinoma cuniculatum; occasionally confused with melanoma if bleeding occurs under the lesion.

Conclusion and key points: these two disorders can be differentiated by paring the warty surface with a razor or scalpel blade. This reveals dark dots (thrombosed vessels) in plantar warts, whereas a pared corn has a smooth shiny pearly focus of keratin.

Comparative features		
Disorder	**Plantar wart (verruca)**	**Plantar corn**
Age	Any, mostly children or young adult	Mostly middle-age onwards
Sex	Either	
Family history	Non-specific	
Sites	Any part of sole of foot	Weight-bearing area of sole, especially forefoot over the metatarsal heads
Symptoms	None, pain on pressure due to hyperkeratosis	Pain on pressure due to hyperkeratosis
Signs common to both	Localized keratotic nodule	
Discriminatory signs	May be painful when squeezed. Dark dots or pinpoint bleeding when pared. Often multiple lesions; may be broad or with adjacent smaller warts	Central shiny pearly area when pared. Usually solitary. Painful on pressure rather than when squeezed
Associated features	May be warts elsewhere	May be abnormal foot shape or posture. Examination of shoes may reveal obvious defects in the sole leading to localized pressure.
Important tests	None	Examine footwear for localizing causes

Further reading:
p. 72, p. 178.

References
Gibbs RC, Boxer MC. Abnormal biomechanics of feet and their causes of hyperkeratoses. *J Am Acad Dermatol* 1982; **6**:1061–9.
Rasmussen KA. Verrucae plantares: symptomatology and epidemiology. *Acta Dermatovener* 1958: **38**(Suppl 39):1–146.

Singh D, Bentley G, Trevino SG. Callosities, corns, and calluses. *BMJ* 1996; **312**:1403–6.

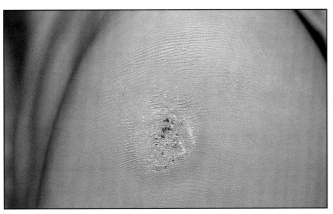

Figure 35.1 *Plantar wart pared to demonstrate dark dots of thrombosed vessels.*

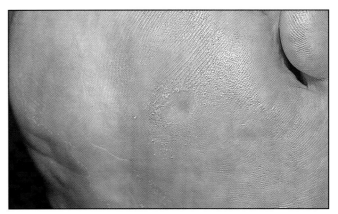

Figure 35.2 *Corn pared to demonstrate central pearly keratin nodule.*

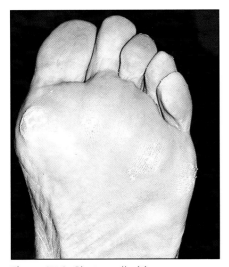

Figure 35.3 *Plantar callosities over metatarsal heads.*

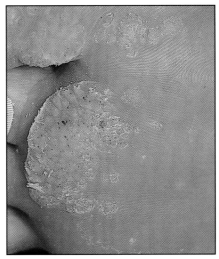

Figure 35.4 *Mosaic warts, showing multiple confluent small warts. Note the black dots of thrombosed vessels.*

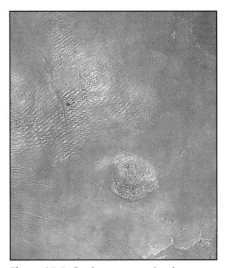

Figure 35.5 *Eccrine poroma, showing a well-circumscribed tender plantar nodule with slightly 'squashed' appearance.*

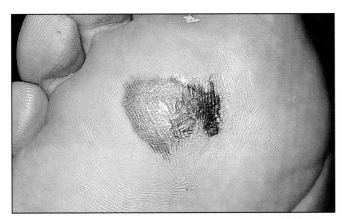

Figure 35.6 *Plantar haematoma, pared to demonstrate old blood clot. Such lesions may be confused with malignant melanoma.*

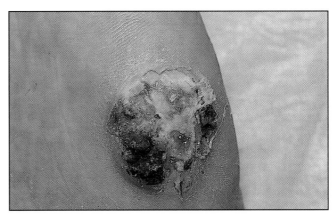

Figure 35.7 *Carcinoma cuniculatum on the sole of the foot: this is a rare type of squamous cell carcinoma which should be suspected if there is a long history of a progressive solitary 'wart', or in elderly patients with an isolated warty plantar nodule(see also Fig. 89.2).*

36 Granuloma annulare v. viral wart (hand or foot site)

Common presenting feature: both disorders may present as localized skin–coloured nodule(s).

Rationale for comparison: both disorders are common on the hands and feet, especially in children. Treatment of the two conditions is different.

Other differential diagnoses: other solitary or multiple discrete nodules on extremities (e.g. corn and/or callosity, eccrine poroma, mastocytoma, dermatofibroma (Fig. 76.3), knuckle pads, acquired digital fibrokeratoma); annular rashes (especially ringworm and sarcoidosis); rarities, such as juvenile fibromatoses.

Conclusion and key points: granuloma annulare (GA) on the hands or feet occurs on the dorsum rather than on the palm or sole, and usually on the hand or foot itself rather than on fingers or toes. By comparison with warts, GA has a smooth and cobblestoned rather than a verrucous or warty surface; although initially papular, lesions of GA become more annular as they enlarge. GA lesions are usually solitary, whereas warts are commonly multiple. Ringworm is also confused with GA; however, it is easily differentiated by the presence of scaling (which indicates epidermal involvement), whereas GA has a smooth surface.

Comparative features		
Disorder	**Granuloma annulare (GA)**	**Viral wart**
Age	Any, mainly children or young adults (in the older age group, consider the possibility of diabetes mellitus)	Any, mainly children or young adults (in adults with new warts, consider the possibility of immunosuppression)
Sex	Female predominance	Either
Family history	Non-specific	
Sites	Usually occurs on the dorsum of the hand or foot, often over bony prominence	Any part of hand or foot, often periungual (p. 178)
Symptoms	None, sometimes tender on direct pressure	Usually painless, may be sore (especially if fissured)
Signs common to both	Localized, skin-coloured (may be pale or slightly yellow) nodule(s) or plaque	
Discriminatory signs	No epidermal component, therefore smooth surface. Often cobblestoned surface, and annular morphology as it expands laterally. Central cleared area is clinically normal or or has a slightly purple or brown colour (post-inflammatory pigmentation)	Surface is rough or warty (but may be influenced by topical therapy or cryotherapy). Black dots due to thrombosed vessels are often visible (Figs. 35.1 and 36.3) and there may be an elevated rim of normal skin in the shape of an acorn cup. Warts are typically multiple lesions; on the foot they are usually plantar, and on the hands the periungual area is a common site (both of these sites are rare for GA).
Associated features	Association with diabetes was thought to be common but is in reality very unusual in the typical young age-group; there is an association between rarer forms of GA (generalized, perforating, or subcutaneous types) and diabetes mellitus.	None
Important tests	In children, tests to detect diabetes mellitus are not indicated unless the patient has relevant symptoms. Urinalysis is adequate in adults.	None

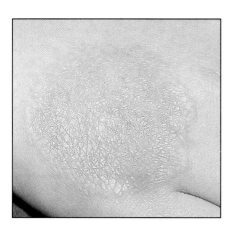

Figure 36.1
Granuloma annulare on hand: this is a broad lesion with typical thickened edge and a rather more cobblestoned centre than found in some lesions.

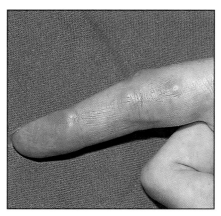

Figure 36.2
Granuloma annulare: showing annular lesions overlying each interphalangeal joint. The proximal lesion has spontaneously flattened around most of the periphery to leave two papular areas; this pattern is especially likely to be confused with warts.

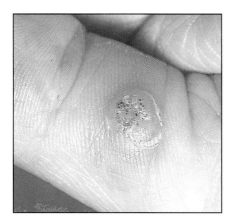

Figure 36.3 *Viral wart on the thumb of a child: this has a verrucous surface which is not a feature of granuloma annulare. Note the black thrombosed vessels.*

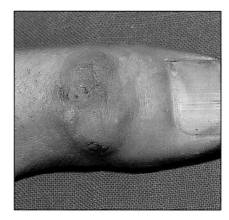

Figure 36.4
Recurrent wart after cryotherapy, showing an annular shape but a less discrete border than occurs in granuloma annulare.

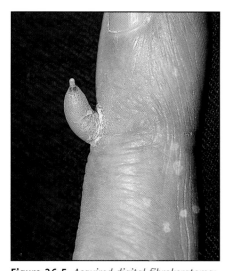

Figure 36.5 *Acquired digital fibrokeratoma: a more elongated lesion with a keratotic tip.*

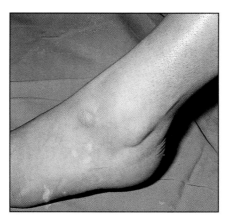

Figure 36.6 *Dorsal foot callosity: these lesions are common and are frictional lesions related to posture when sitting (they are often symmetrical).*

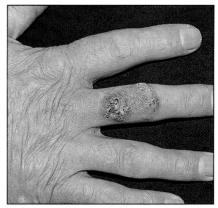

Figure 36.7 *Fish-tank granuloma (*Mycobacterium marinum *infection): this may initially resemble a wart but is more crusted and enlarges rapidly.*

Further reading:
p. 70, p. 78, p. 178.

References
Joseph AB, Herr B. Finger calluses in bulimia. *Am J Psychiatr* 1985: **5**:655.
Cox NH, Finlay AY. Crossed leg callosities. *Acta Dermatovenereol* 1985; 65:292–5.

Guberman D, Lichtenstein DA, Vardy DA. Knuckle pads—a forgotten skin condition. Report of a case and review of the literature. *Cutis* 1996; **57**:241–2.
Muhlbauer JE. Granuloma annulare. *J Am Acad Dermatol* 1980; **3**:217–30.

Common presenting features: rash on dorsum of hands, with fragile skin and blisters and erosions.

Rationale for comparison: importance of correct treatment; topical corticosteroids will aggravate the skin fragility of porphyria cutanea tarda, which requires systemic therapy and avoidance of provoking factors.

Other differential diagnoses: photodermatoses; pseudoporphyria (due to naproxen, nalidixic acid and other drugs); sunbed-induced skin fragility; simple repetitive injury; bullous plant contact reactions; other porphyrias (variegate, erythropoietic protoporphyria);

epidermolysis bullosa acquisita.

Conclusion and key points: PCT should be considered in any apparently eczematous rash with undue skin fragility affecting sun-exposed skin. Erythropoietic protoporphyria is usually easily differentiated by its early childhood onset and by a history of pain or a burning sensation immediately after sunlight exposure. The rash of variegate porphyria is indistinguisthable from PCT, but may be suspected from the associated systemic symptoms. PCT is uncommon but often characteristic in retrospect, and is an important diagnosis because of the systemic implications and fundamentally different treatment.

Comparative features		
Disorder	**Porphyria cutanea tarda (PCT)**	**Hand eczema**
Age	Usual onset in middle-age	Any
Sex	Male predominance	Either
Family history	May be sporadic or autosomal dominant, in which case family history is positive	Non-specific
Sites	Dorsal surface of hands, may affect face	Confusion with PCT is most likely if eczema is confined to the dorsum of the hands, but in most cases it affects other parts of the hands also.
Symptoms	Soreness due to erosions. The photosensitive aspect is not usually appreciated by the patient.	Itch
Signs common to both	Scaling, crusting	
Discriminatory signs	Unilocular blisters (usually 0.5–1 cm diameter), atrophic scars which may be hyperpigmented, milia, skin fragility and erosions, hypertrichosis (usually most apparent on the temples)	Eczematous changes; background erythema, scaling, lichenification, and fissures. Pompholyx eczema causes small blisters which are multilocular and usually on palm, border of hand, sides of fingers
Associated features	Metabolic abnormalities (see below). Typically history of excess alcohol, or other drug triggers (oestrogens, halogenated aromatic hydrocarbons). A history of abdominal or neurological symptoms suggests variegate porphyria rather than PCT.	There may be eczematous nail changes (these are not a feature of PCT), or eczema at other body sites.
Important tests	Porphyrin screen. In PCT the main abnormality is elevation of urinary uroporphyrins: these should be formally measured but may be detected as a simple screening method by fluorescence (see Fig. 37.6). In variegate porphyria, the major porphyrin excretion is faecal, and stool porphyrins should be measured. Glucose, ferritin, and liver transaminase levels are all commonly elevated.	Patch tests may be required; +/- phototesting

Further reading:
p. 32, p. 40, p. 76, p. 106, p. 114, p. 116, p. 142.

References
Bickers DR. Porphyrias. In: Wojnarowska F, Briggaman RA (eds). *Management of blistering disorders*. Chapman & Hall, London, 1990:277–88.
Grossman ME, Poh-Fitzpatrick MB. Porphyria cutanea tarda. Diagnosis, management, and differentiation from other hepatic porphyrias. *Dermatol Clinics* 1986; **4**:297–309.
Higgins EM, du Vivier AW. Cutaneous disease and alcohol misuse. *Br Med Bull* 1994; **50**:85–98.

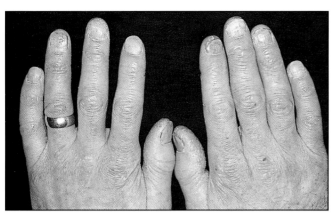

Figure 37.1 *Eczema affecting dorsal hands and fingers, showing diffuse erythema, scaling, fissures, and nail changes.*

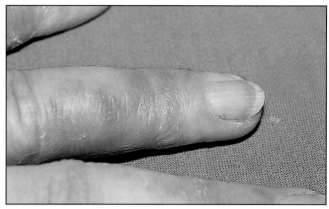

Figure 37.2 *Eczema (close-up), showing erythema and fine scaling on the dorsum of fingers.*

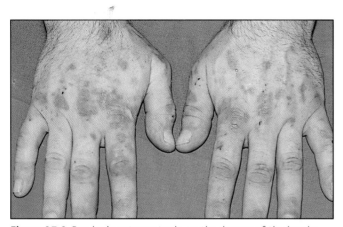

Figure 37.3 *Porphyria cutanea tarda on the dorsum of the hands: there are scattered discrete lesions rather than the more diffuse pattern seen in eczemas.*

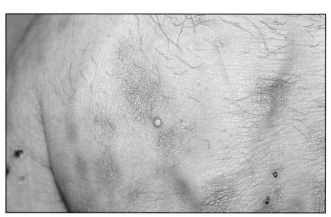

Figure 37.4 *Porphyria cutanea tarda (close-up), showing healing erosions, pigmented depressed scars, and a milium.*

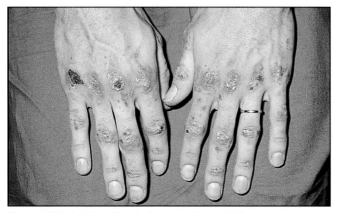

Figure 37.5 *Epidermolysis bullosa acquisita: this is an uncommon bullous disorder, in this case associated with Crohn's disease. Milia are prominent in this example.*

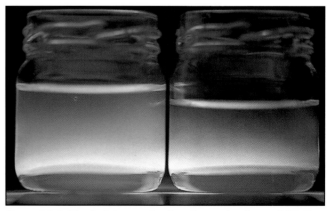

Figure 37.6 *Wood's light examination of a routine (non-acidified) urine sample in a patient with porphyria cutanea tarda: this demonstrates prominent pink fluorescence compared with a normal control.*

38 Chronic irritant v. allergic hand eczema

Common presenting feature: itchy eczematous eruption.

Rationale for comparison: these two cannot always be differentiated by history or clinical differences and may coexist, as irritants may perpetuate either type.

Other differential diagnoses: psoriasis of hands (p. 58, Fig. 29.1); atopic eczema (as this is typically aggravated by irritants); other specific patterns of eczema (hyperkeratotic, discoid, pompholyx); scabies; fungal infection (p. 62, Fig. 31.2); secondary ('id') eruptions usually related to severe tinea pedis; dermatomyositis.

Conclusion and key points: the history of onset or timing of the rash, and its apparent relationship to likely irritants or allergens, is usually more important than the clinical appearance. In the early stages, irritant hand eczema is typically limited to the web spaces or adjacent dorsum of hands, or under rings. However, this is not specific. For example, a rash under rings may be due to trapped irritants or to metal allergy, and allergens in liquid form affect the same distribution as irritant liquids.

Comparative features

Disorder	Chronic irritant hand eczema	Chronic allergic hand eczema
Age	Any	
Sex	Female predominance	Occupational causes are more common in men
Family history	Non-specific. Atopic patients are vulnerable to irritant hand eczema, however, even in the absence of recent atopic dermatitis at typical sites.	Non-specific
Sites	Often starts under rings, in webspaces or on the dorsum of hands, but may be limited to sites such as fingertips (e.g. in cooks)	May be specifically related to the allergen contact site (e.g. fingertips due to handling plants or foods, cut-off at wrists due to rubber glove use), but may be non-specific
Symptoms	Itch, soreness if fissured. Allergic types may fluctuate more in degree of severity.	
Signs common to both	Chronic eczema (dry scaling, erythema, fissures); possibly with vesicles during acute exacerbations	
Discriminatory signs	None specific	None specific, unless clear relationship to pattern of a contact allergen (e.g. sharp cut-off at wrists related to rubber glove use)
Associated features	May be atopic skin or respiratory symptoms, e.g. xerosis, dermatitis	May be evidence of contact with the same allergen at other sites (e.g. patients with hand dermatitis due to nickel may also have reactions to earrings, jeans studs, rings etc.)
Important tests	Patch test to exclude contact allergy unless there is a clear irritant on basis of history and response to emollients and hand protection	Patch testing
Relative frequency	Common	Less common

Further reading:
p. 22, p. 32, p. 38, p. 58.

References
Adams RM. Patch testing. A recapitulation. *J Am Acad Dermatol* 1981; **5**:629–43.
Adams RM. *Occupational skin disease*, 2nd edn. Philadelphia, WB Saunders, 1990.
Fisher AA. *Contact dermatitis*, 3rd edn. Philadelphia, Lea and Febinger, 1986:258–82.

Meding B, Swanbeck G. Predictive factors for hand eczema. *Contact Dermatitis* 1990; **23**:154–61.
Rystedt I. Factors influencing the occurrence of hand eczema in adults with a history of atopic dermatitis in childhood. *Contact Dermatitis* 1985; **12**:185–91.

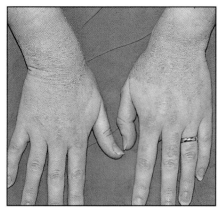

Figure 38.1 *Diffuse eczema of dorsal hands and fingers, due to contact allergy to rubber gloves. Note the cut-off at the wrists.*

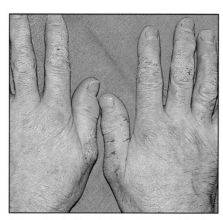

Figure 38.2 *Chronic irritant dermatitis of hands with fissuring: a glove allergy could not be excluded on clinical grounds.*

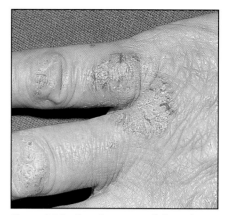

Figure 38.3 *Chronic eczema of the web space: an irritant cause was likely but the patient had a strong positive patch test to lanolin (wool alcohols), which was a constituent of her hand cream.*

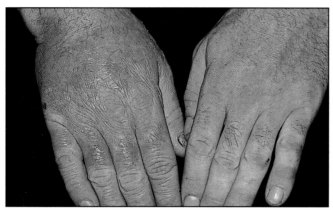

Figure 38.4 *Tinea incognito: there is fungal infection masked by use of topical corticosteroids. Always consider fungal infection in any asymmetrical 'eczema'.*

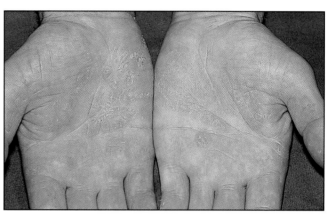

Figure 38.5 *Symmetrical hyperkeratotic palmar dermatitis: this is an endogenous pattern.*

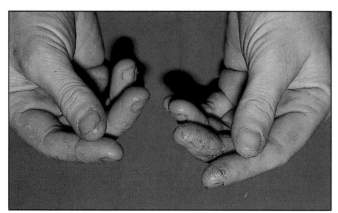

Figure 38.6 *Fingertip eczema in a cook: this is highly suggestive of allergy to foods (typically garlic). The non-dominant hand and index to ring fingers are characteristically affected, as these hold the food whilst the dominant hand holds a knife or other kitchen implement.*

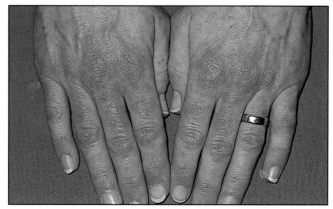

Figure 38.7 *Dermatomyositis: the cutaneous features may resemble eczema, but the lesions are typically violaceous, have a streaky pattern on the dorsum of fingers, and include nail fold and cuticle involvement.*

39 Squamous cell carcinoma v. actinic keratosis

Common presenting feature: hyperkeratotic lesion or 'cutaneous horn'.

Rationale for comparison: different intensity of treatment required.

Other differential diagnoses: other localized keratotic lesions, e.g. keratoacanthoma (p. 52), viral wart, seborrhoeic keratosis (p. 162, Fig. 28.5); Bowen's disease (p. 156, Fig. 28.1); less common tumours, e.g. atypical fibroxanthoma.

Conclusion and key points: simple actinic keratoses are usually multiple, have a hard spiky keratinous surface, and are not indurated or thickened at the base. Treatment of actinic keratoses includes emollients, cryotherapy, 5-fluorouracil, curettage, and sometimes excision. Squamous cell carcinoma are generally solitary and have a fleshy indurated base, and are best treated by excision or radiotherapy. In some cases, thicker (so-called 'hypertrophic') actinic keratoses may be difficult to differentiate from squamous cell carcinoma (SCC) and may need excision. This diagnostic comparison also applies to other sun-exposed skin on face or limbs.

Comparative features		
Disorder	**Squamous cell carcinoma (SCC)**	**Actinic keratosis**
Age	Middle-age onwards	
Sex	Male predominance	
Family history	Non-specific	
Sites	Any habitually sun-exposed site	
Symptoms	Usually none, may be painful, may catch on cuffs of clothing	Usually none unless catching on clothing
Signs common to both	Localized hard hyperkeratotic lesion or keratin horn	
Discriminatory signs	Fleshy base. May have moist or crusted surface rather than formed keratosis. Concurrent regional lymphadenopathy is rare but confirms malignancy.	Formed keratosis, no fleshy epidermal base
Associated features	Both are associated with other evidence of solar damage, and most patients with an SCC will also have actinic keratoses.	Both are common in immunosuppressed patients (especially post-transplant surgery).
Important tests	Excision and histological examination	None unless diagnostic concern

Further reading:
p. 20, p. 40, p. 52, p. 54, p. 154, p. 156.

References
Kwa RE, Campana K, Moy RL. Biology of cutaneous squamous cell carcinoma. *J Am Acad Dermatol* 1992; **26**:1–26.
Marks R, Selwood TS. Solar keratoses. The association with erythemal ultraviolet radiation in Australia. *Cancer* 1985; **56**:2332–6.

Schwartz RA. Premalignant keratinocytic neoplasms. *J Am Acad Dermatol* 1996; **35**:223–42.
Sober AJ, Burnstein JM. Precursors of skin cancer. *Cancer* 1995; **75**:645–50.

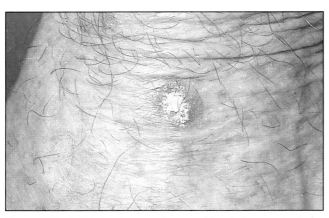

Figure 39.1 *Actinic keratoses on dorsum of hand: there are typical discrete lesions with spiky keratin horn.*

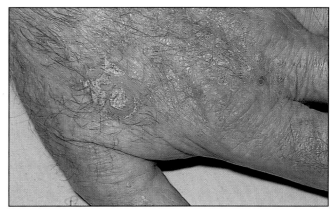

Figure 39.2 *Squamous cell carcinoma on dorsum of hand, on a background of extensive actinic keratoses. Note the fleshy basal thickening.*

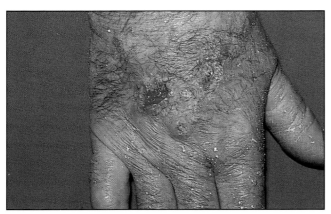

Figure 39.3 *Squamous cell carcinoma of hand, showing a broad lesion with nodularity and ulceration. The white dots are paint from the patient's occupation.*

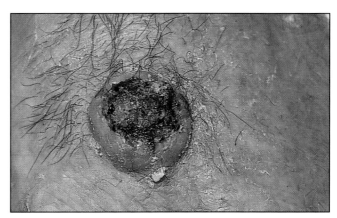

Figure 39.4 *Squamous cell carcinoma, showing a larger and more indurated lesion than that in Fig. 39.3 with central crusting rather than a formed keratosis.*

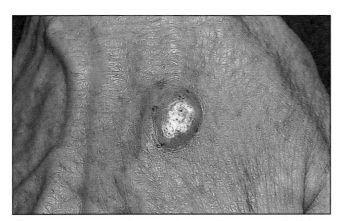

Figure 39.5 *Keratoacanthoma on the hand (see also p. 52). This demonstrates the clinical difficulty in distinction from SCC.*

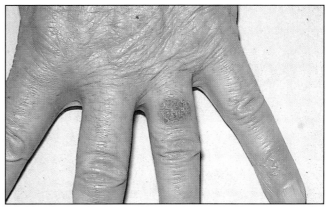

Figure 39.6 *Bowen's disease: the dorsum of the proximal phalanx is a moderately common site, and lesions are often resistant to treatment here.*

Common presenting feature: scattered rash, often following upper respiratory tract infection.

Rationale for comparison: guttate psoriasis usually takes about 2 months to resolve, whereas a viral exanthem usually settles in 1–2 weeks. Accurate diagnosis is therefore helpful in order to give appropriate explanation, and also because specific treaments are available to accelerate the resolution of psoriasis.

Other differential diagnoses: drug eruption (p. 104); pityriasis versicolor (p. 90); pityriasis rosea; pityriasis rubra pilaris; tinea corporis; Gianotti–Crosti syndrome.

Conclusion and key points: in the very early stages, distinguishing between these two disorders may be difficult. Guttate psoriasis lesions are more keratotic, whereas a viral eruption has finer or absent scaling. Peeling of the skin after a viral exanthem is common, but also occurs after streptococcal infections or some drug eruptions. Illustrations of different patterns of viral exanthem may be seen on p. 105. Topical corticosteroids may reduce itch and erythema in either of these disorders, but the spectrum of possible treatment is greater for guttate psoriasis, and includes treatment with ultraviolet light, tars, vitamin-D analogues, and/or dithranol preparations.

Comparative features		
Disorder	**Guttate psoriasis**	**Viral exanthem**
Age	Child or young adult. Some older adults with established psoriasis have relapses with a guttate pattern.	Any
Sex	Either	
Family history	May be positive for psoriasis	May be familial (or school or work colleagues) with sore throat or viral symptoms
Sites	Mainly truncal	
Symptoms	None, itch	
Signs common to both	Scattered small plaques; fairly abrupt onset	
Discriminatory signs	Hyperkeratosis (especially focal scalp hyperkeratosis); lesions are often rather papular. The Koebner reaction is common in eruptive psoriasis.	Finer scaling, often at the periphery of lesions. These are usually broader patches than in guttate psoriasis, often oval rather than round lesions, and more likely to be confluent. Some specific identifiable patterns may occur, e.g. herald patch of pityriasis rosea, umbilicated papules of Gianotti-Crosti syndrome.
Associated features	Typically occurs 10 days after streptococcal sore throat, so patients may still have enlarged tonsils. Psoriasis may be present at typical sites (knees, elbows, scalp), with nail changes, etc., but this is uncommon in typical young age-group patients.	Preceding illness is usually more 'flu-like' rather than a simple upper respiratory tract infection, and often with a shorter interval between the trigger and development of rash (therefore patients may have concurrent pyrexia, lymphadenopathy, palatal purpura etc.).
Important tests	Look for evidence of current of preceding streptococcal infection (bacteriology swab from tonsils, blood for antistreptolysin titre).	Viral titres are occasionally positive. Throat swab. Monospot test

Further reading:
p. 2, p. 82, p. 102, p. 104.

References
Chuang TY, *et al.* Pityriasis rosea in Rochester, Minnesota, 1969–78. *J Am Acad Dermatol* 1982; **7**:80–9.
Griffiths CE. Psoriasis. I. Pathogenesis. *J Am Acad Dermatol* 1992; **27**:98–101.
Taieb A, *et al.* Gianotti–Crosti syndrome: a study of 26 cases. *Br J Dermatol* 1986; **115**:49–59.
Telfer NR, *et al.* The role of streptococcal infection in the initiation of guttate psoriasis. *Arch Dermatol* 1992; **128**:39–42.

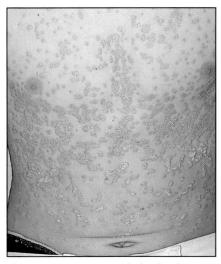

Figure 40.1 *Guttate psoriasis, showing typical truncal distribution of discrete, tiny, scaly plaques.*

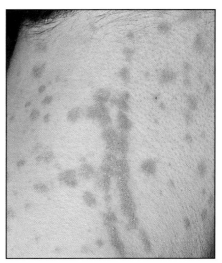

Figure 40.2 *Guttate psoriasis with lesions localized to a site of minor injury (Koebner reaction).*

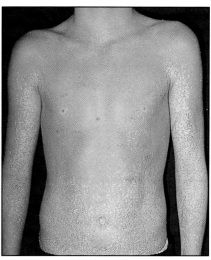

Figure 40.3 *Pityriasis rubra pilaris: this is a disorder which is rather psoriasiform, but often develops more acutely over a period of a few weeks, as in this case. The rather more orange colour is typical of Pityriasis rubra pilaris.*

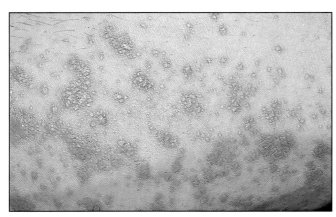

Figure 40.4 *Eruptive lichen planus: this may simulate a viral exanthem. Lesions are typically rather purple in colour and shiny on the surface. Although not shown here, they may demonstrate a Koebner reaction as in guttate psoriasis.*

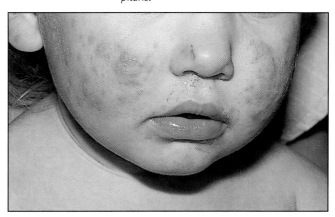

Figure 40.5 *Gianotti–Crosti syndrome, a post-viral rash (most commonly due to Epstein–Barr virus) which lasts a few weeks in children, typically affecting face, arms, and knees. Individual lesions are umbilicated papules.*

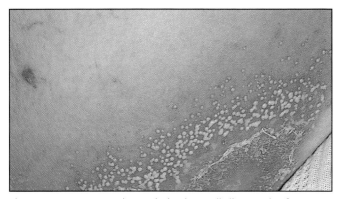

Figure 40.6 *Acute pustular psoriasis: the small silvery scale of guttate psoriasis is occasionally mistakenly thought to be pustular, but true pustular psoriasis is a much more aggressive disease. It may be confused with pustular viral lesions such as those in varicella (see Fig. 40.7).*

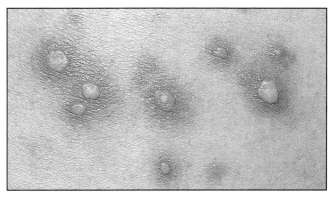

Figure 40.7 *Varicella. Pustular lesions of chickenpox may cause diagnostic confusion in adults.*

Plaque psoriasis v. parapsoriasis

Common presenting feature: variably itchy, scaly erythematous plaques.

Rationale for comparison: parapsoriasis often responds better to ultraviolet therapies (UVA, PUVA) than to topical corticosteroids. The distinction from psoriasis is important as parapsoriasis is worsened by most other topical psoriasis treatments, and also because large plaque types may be premalignant (see mycosis fungoides, p. 84, Fig. 42.3).

Other differential diagnoses: specific types of dermatitis (e.g. seborrhoeic dermatitis); tinea corporis; pityriasis versicolor (p. 90, Fig. 45.1); mycosis fungoides (p. 84,); Darier's disease.

Conclusion and key points: the most frequent types of parapsoriasis can generally be differentiated by their digitate pattern on the flanks, uniform size of lesions, and relatively fine scale and mild erythema compared with psoriasis. Unlike with psoriasis, nail lesions do not occur, scalp involvement is very unlikely, and there is no particular tendency for lesions to occur on elbows or knees. Buttocks and flanks are often involved, but there is no specific localization to flexures as can occur in psoriasis. Parapsoriasis is most likely to be confused with more common dermatitic processes.

Comparative features		
Disorder	**Plaque psoriasis**	**Parapsoriasis**
Age	Any age; peak onset is in young adults	Adult, very rare in children
Sex	Either	
Family history	May be positive	Non-specific
Sites	Any. Typical sites are extensor aspects of elbows and knees, scalp, flexures, nails (none of which are likely sites for parapsoriasis). It is unusual to have significant trunk lesions without lesions at some of the more typical sites also.	Mainly affects the flanks, buttocks, and relatively light-shielded areas of limbs, e.g. inner aspect of upper arm
Symptoms	None, itch	None, mild itch
Signs common to both	Scaling erythematous plaques	
Discriminatory signs	Plaques are more thickened and erythematous, with a prominent silvery scaling component. They are usually more varied in size and scattered in distribution compared with parapsoriasis.	Lesions are flat, pink rather than red, and have a fine branny scale. They are typically of relatively uniform size, often with oval or digitate shape (especially on the flanks). Finely wrinkled skin or mild poikiloderma (atrophy, telangiectasia, and pigmentation) is common.
Associated features	Lesions at other sites, e.g. scalp and limbs; may be nail changes (p. 174) or joint disease	None usually, but other lymphoctic infiltrates (e.g. lymphomatoid papulosis or poikiloderma) may coexist
Important tests	None	Apart from mild cases with a typical digitate pattern, a skin biopsy is often performed as large plaque size variants may be a precursor of mycosis fungoides, a cutaneous T-cell lymphoma

Further reading:
pp. 58–64, p. 80, p. 84, p. 102, p. 118.

References

Hu CH, Winkelmann RK. Digitate dermatosis. A new look at symmetrical small plaque parapsoriasis. *Arch Dermatol* 1973; **107**:65–9.

Kikuchi A, *et al.* Parapsoriasis en plaque: its potential for progression to malignant lymphoma. *J Am Acad Dermatol* 1993; **29**:419–22.

Lambert WC, Everett MA. The nosology of parapsoriasis. *J Am Acad Dermatol* 1981; **5**:373–95.

Smith NP. Histologic criteria for early diagnosis of cutaneous T-cell lymphoma. *Dermatol Clinics* 1994; **12**:315–22.

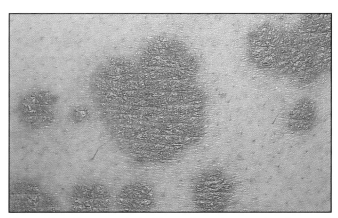

Figure 41.1 *Plaque psoriasis (close-up): erythema and scaling are more prominent than in parapsoriasis.*

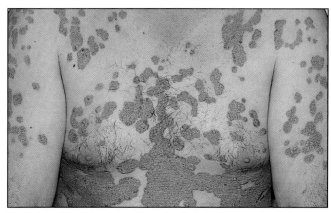

Figure 41.2 *Psoriasis, showing scattered distribution, irregularly sized, and relatively inflammatory plaques.*

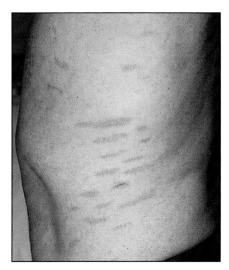

Figure 41.3
Parapsoriasis: this variant, called digitate dermatosis, is a clinically characteristic benign pattern and typically affects the flanks.

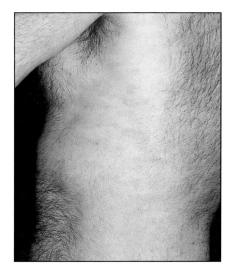

Figure 41.4
Parapsoriasis: this rather vaguer pattern is more typical of the disease. Flank involvement is common: note the paler colour and finer scaling than are found in psoriasis.

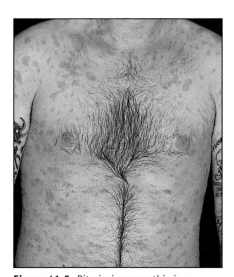

Figure 41.5 *Pityriasis rosea: this is a clinically characteristic self-limiting exanthem with oval shaped lesions and peripheral scale. It is eruptive and presumed to have an infective cause.*

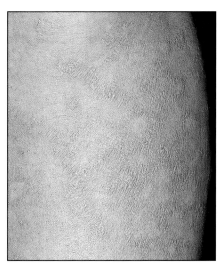

Figure 41.6 *A patchy diffuse eczema: this is less aggressive and more confluent than discoid eczema. This pattern of eczema may be confused with parapsoriasis.*

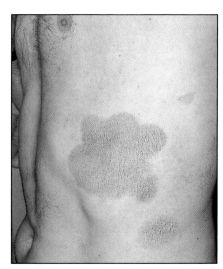

Figure 41.7 *Mycosis fungoides: this was a low grade process preceded by a prolonged and relatively static phase classified as large plaque parapsoriasis.*

Common presenting feature: scaly erythematous plaques.

Rationale for comparison: these disorders have different treatments and prognosis. Psoriasis is a common inflammatory dermatosis which has a variable course but is mild in most affected individuals. Mycosis fungoides (MF) is a cutaneous T-cell lymphoma which is usually controllable in most patients but potentially has a progressive course and may cause death from systemic involvement. Psoriasis is usually treated topically in the vast majority of patients, whereas MF is usually treated with PUVA and sometimes requires radiotherapy, topical or systemic cytotoxic agents, or extracorporeal phototherapy.

Other differential diagnoses: eczemas (discoid and seborrhoeic eczemas may be confused with early MF; diffuse long-standing atopic eczema may be difficult to differentiate clinically from erythrodermic MF); pityriasis rubra pilaris; drug eruptions; parapsoriasis; tinea corporis; chronic photosensitivity dermatitis/actinic reticuloid.

Conclusion and key points: MF can usually be differentiated clinically by the appearance of different shades of colour and different thickness of lesions; these produce an appearance of superimposed lesions. In psoriasis, lesions are generally discrete or coalesce by radial expansion, in which case they merge to form a solitary larger lesion. Psoriasis has a greater degree of hyperkeratosis and silvery scale. In erythrodermic patients, it may be impossible to differentiate these disorders without histological examination of a skin biopsy.

Comparative features		
Disorder	**Extensive psoriasis**	**Mycosis fungoides (MF)**
Age	Any, onset usually in young adults	Mostly > 40 yr
Sex	Either	Male predominance
Family history	May be positive	Non-specific
Sites	Mainly limbs if mild. There is potential for confusion, however, if the distribution is mainly truncal or if lesions are confluent or erythrodermic.	Lesions occur mainly on the trunk or buttocks initially, but may eventually affect any site including palms, soles, and scalp.
Symptoms	Itch, variable	Itch, usually severe
Signs common to both	Erythematous scaling plaques; both are causes of generalized erythroderma	
Discriminatory signs	Sharply defined discrete lesions, which may be annular due to radial spread and central clearing. These are typically variable with time, and have silvery psoriatic scale pattern. There may be typical psoriasis at other sites (scalp, elbows, knees, nails) or other clues such as areas of Koebner reaction (Fig. 40.2).	Lesions are less well defined, and have finer scale. They may be annular or arciform in shape but neat rings with central clearing are less common than in psoriasis. Typically lesions have the appearance of different shades superimposed on each other. There is usually slow progression in severity; nodules, ulceration, and alopecia occur in advanced disease.
Associated features	Psoriatic arthritis may be a clue. Lymphadenopathy may occur in patients with extensive psoriasis, particularly if erythrodermic.	There may be associated lymphadenopathy. Nails are usually normal but can be affected, especially in erythroderma (pitting is not a feature).
Important tests	None unless ill or erythrodermic	Skin biopsy (may require special immunocytochemical stains). Screen for systemic disease and atypical circulating lymphocytes in progressive MF.

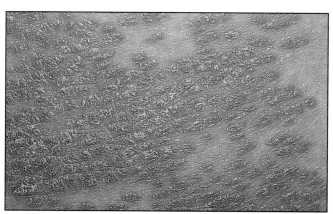

Figure 42.1 *Psoriasis: the degree of erythema and silvery scaling is usually fairly constant for all lesions (compare with psoriasis in Figs. 41.1, 41.2, and with mycosis fungoides in Figs 42.3, 42.4).*

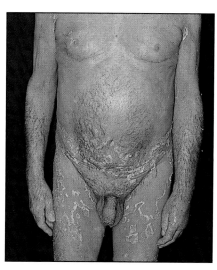

Figure 42.2
Erythroderma, in this case, due to psoriasis. Unless there is a clear previous history, or specific features such as psoriatic nail pits (p. 174), the cause of erythroderma may be difficult to determine. It is important to do this because of the different treatments which may be required.

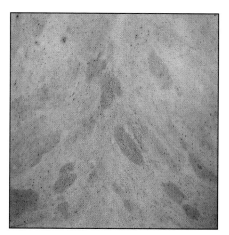

Figure 42.3 *Mycosis fungoides: note the coexistence of lesions of various shades of pink and red.*

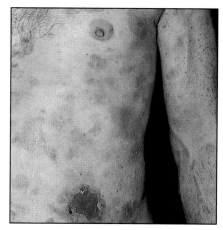

Figure 42.4 *Mycosis fungoides: there are more advanced lesions with some early ulceration.*

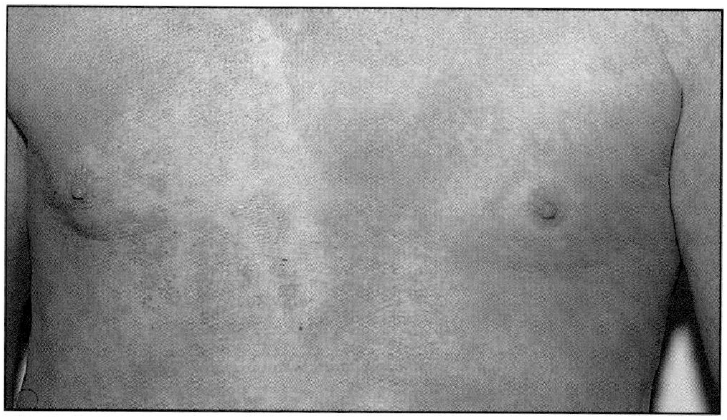

Figure 42.5 *Pityriasis rubra pilaris: the erythrodermic form is characterized by rapid cephalocaudal spread and by isolated 'islands' of sparing (see also Fig. 40.3).*

Causes of erythroderma	
Eczemas (atopic, contact, seborrheic)	40%
Psoriasis	30%
Drug eruptions (allopurinol, penicillins, anticonvulsants, sulphonamides)	15%
Cutaneous lymphomas/ Sezary syndrome	10%
Others (pityriasis rubra pilaris, some ichthoses, infestations, dermatophytosis)	5%

Further reading:
pp. 58–64, p. 82, p. 102, p. 118.

References
Holloway KB, Flowers FP, Ramos–Caro FA. Therapeutic alternatives in cutaneous T-cell lymphoma. *J Am Acad Dermatol* 1992; **27**:367–78.
Lorincz AL. Cutaneous T-cell lymphoma (mycosis fungoides). *Lancet* 1996; **347**:871–6.

Wieselthier JS, Koh HK. Sezary syndrome: diagnosis, prognosis, and critical review of treatment options. *J Am Acad Dermatol* 1990; **22**:381–401.

43 Discoid eczema v. superficial basal cell carcinoma

Common presenting feature: localized crusting plaque on trunk.

Rationale for comparison: superficial basal cell carcinoma (BCC) is commonly not diagnosed until it has been present for some years. It requires surgical treatment or radiotherapy rather than anti-inflammatory treatment.

Other differential diagnoses: psoriasis; tinea (ringworm); seborrhoeic keratosis (especially flat type, see Fig. 67.5); Bowen's disease, p. 156; discoid lupus erythematosus; Paget's disease, Fig. 49.2.

Conclusion and key points: superficial BCC is generally easily diagnosed once suspected. The lesions are usually solitary or few in number, cause few symptoms, slowly enlarge with no response to antifungal or corticosteroid creams, and have a characteristic shiny surface and narrow raised border. Distinction from eczema or ringworm is very rarely a problem in dermatology clinics, but these conditions may be confused by non-specialists.

Comparative features		
Disorder	**Discoid eczema**	**Superficial basal cell carcinoma (BCC)**
Age	Mostly >40 yr	
Sex	Either	Male predominance
Family history	Non-specific	
Sites	Any; most confusion arises on the trunk, which is the most frequent site for superficial BCC	
Symptoms	Itch. Lesions are variable in time and site affected, and may completely resolve.	None; minor irritation in larger lesions if crusted. Lesions slowly enlarge in diameter.
Signs common to both	Discoid patch with some surface crust	
Discriminatory signs	Usually prominent erythema and may be vesiculation, weeping and marked crusting. Fairly well defined but not a sharp border. Usually multiple	Superficial BCCs have a shiny or waxy appearance, often with some pigment variation. They are usually solitary or few in number. The typical sign, best seen with the skin stretched, is a narrow (approx. 1 mm) raised wavy border, which provides a sharp distinction from adjacent skin. Larger lesions may have nodular or ulcerated areas.
Associated features	Usually affects lower limbs also	Occasionally evidence of arsenic ingestion, especially if multiple lesions (palmar keratoses)
Important tests	None	Biopsy and histology
Treatment	Strong topical corticosteroid +/– antibiotic or antiseptic	Excise, curette, cryotherapy (some), radiotherapy (some)

Further reading:
p. 20, p. 40, p. 46, p. 48, p. 98, p. 134, p. 154, p. 156.

References
Florin EH, Kolbusz RV, Goldberg LH. Basal cell carcinoma simulating eczematous dermatitis. *Cutis* 1994; **54**:197–8.

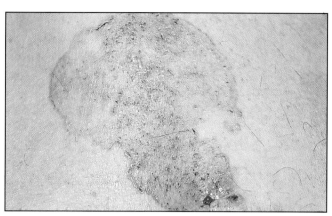

Figure 43.1 *Superficial basal cell carcinoma with a typical irregular narrow elevated border.*

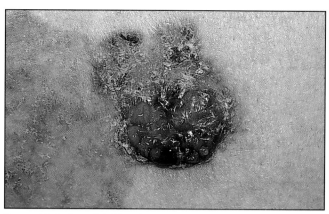

Figure 43.2 *Superficial basal cell carcinoma with a more nodular pigmented component. Some degree of pigmentation is common in this morphology of basal cell carcinoma.*

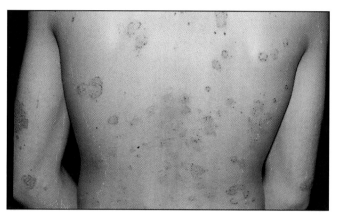

Figure 43.3 *Discoid eczema: lesions are often similar in size to superficial basal cell carcinomas at presentation, and may be of similar colour, but are typically larger and more profuse (compare with Fig. 43.4).*

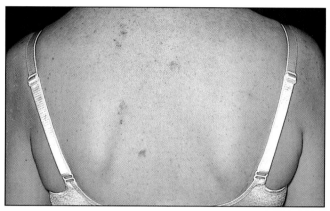

Figure 43.4 *Scattered small basal cell carcinomas on the upper back in a young woman: a larger superficial basal cell carcinoma on her chest had been present for several years (compare with Fig. 43.3).*

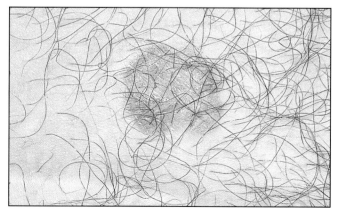

Figure 43.5 *Bowen's disease in the pubic area, treated for ringworm, then as eczema for three years.*

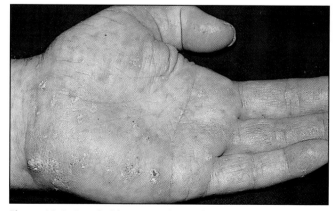

Figure 43.6 *Arsenical keratoses: these reflect ingestion of arsenic several decades previously when it was commonly prescribed as a tonic. These lesions are not uncommon in patients with multiple basal cell carcinomas or multiple lesions of Bowen's disease. The index finger was amputated to treat squamous cell carcinoma.*

44   Acne v. pityrosporum folliculitis

Common presenting feature: papulopustular rash on the trunk, especially the back.

Rationale for comparison: pityrosporum folliculitis is a common, and readily identifiable, cause of 'antibiotic-resistant' acne which in fact requires anti-yeast treatment.

Other differential diagnoses: bacterial folliculitis; keratosis pilaris (p. 132); pustular exanthems and drug eruptions (lithium, phenytoin, halides, isoniazid, corticosteroids).

Conclusion and key points: pityrosporum folliculitis of the trunk is fairly common, particularly in the late teens and in young adults in whom it may be confused with acne. As either disorder may affect this age-group, there is the additional diagnostic complication that the two conditions may coexist. *Pityrosporum* infection produces an extensive but relatively monomorphic picture of papules and pustules affecting the entire back; by contrast, acne produces more mixed lesions including blackheads, nodules, cysts, and scarring, which predominantly affect the upper back.

Comparative features		
Disorder	**Acne**	**Pityrosporum folliculitis**
Age	Early teens to early 20s	Late teens to 50s
Sex	Either	
Family history	Non-specific	
Sites	Mainly upper back and central chest; typically also affects the face	Usually the whole of the back; sometimes scattered lesions on chest; occasionally some facial lesions
Symptoms	Some lesions may be tender.	None, itch
Signs common to both	Papules and pustules on the back and/or the chest	
Discriminatory signs	Presence of varied lesions of acne, which include blackheads, whiteheads, nodules, cysts, scars on the upper back. Pustules are usually 2–5 mm in diameter.	Essentially monomorphic lesions (papules and small 1–2 mm diameter pustules), widely distributed over the whole of the back
Associated features	Acne at other sites, especially the face	Typical lack of response to prolonged courses of antibiotics. There may be signs of other *Pityrosporum* yeast disorders, such as dandruff or seborrhoeic dermatitis.
Important tests	None	*Pityrosporum* yeasts may be visible on skin scrapings from pustular lesions, but are very difficult to culture in the laboratory; diagnosis is primarily clinical.
Therapeutic note	Antibiotics will help acne but have no beneficial effect on pityrosporum folliculitis, which is usually treated with imidazole or triazole antifungal agents. Both disorders may respond to oral retinoids as these reduce sebum production and therefore *Pityrosporum* yeasts, which live in follicular sebum, are reduced in number as a secondary effect. However, in pityrosporum folliculitis, this approach is unnecessary, expensive, and may be followed by rapid relapse in some individuals.	

Further reading:
p. 34, p. 36, p. 90.

References
Back O, Faergermann J, Hornqvist R. Pityrosporum folliculitis. A common disease of the young and middle-aged. *J Am Acad Dermatol* 1985; **12**:56–61.

Ford GP, Ive FA, Midgley G. Pityrosporum folliculitis and ketoconazole. *Br J Dermatol* 1982; **109**:691–5.

Hay RJ. Antifungal therapy of yeast infections. *J Am Acad Dermatol* 1994; **31**:56–9.

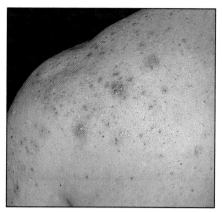

Figure 44.1 *Acne on the back demonstrating the distribution (mainly upper trunk) and the larger, more variable and inflamed lesions than found in pityrosporum folliculitis.*

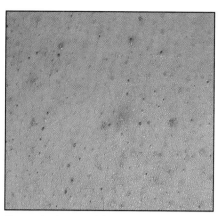

Figure 44.2 *Acne (close-up) demonstrating comedones. These do not occur in pityrosporum folliculitis.*

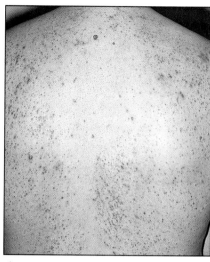

Figure 44.3 *Pityrosporum folliculitis, a relatively severe example, demonstrating the extent and monomorphic nature of the rash, which extends down to the waistline.*

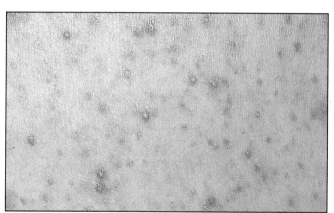

Figure 44.4 *Pityrosporum folliculitis (close-up): this demonstrates the rather monomorphic papules and pustules without comedones or nodules.*

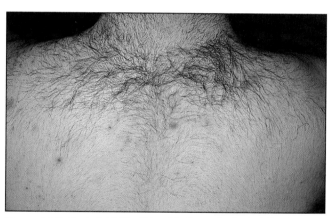

Figure 44.5 *Bacterial folliculitis: affecting only the hair-bearing area of the upper back.*

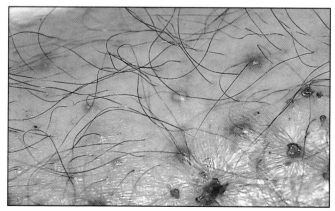

Figure 44.6 *Bacterial folliculitis (close-up): the pustules are larger and more inflammatory than in pityrosporum folliculitis.*

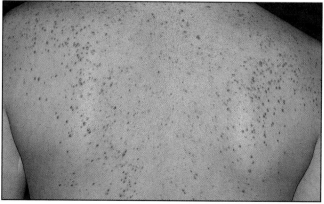

Figure 44.7 *Steroid acne: usually pustular, but again very monomorphic compared with 'ordinary' acne.*

45 Pityriasis versicolor v. vitiligo

Common presenting feature: scattered depigmented patches.

Rationale for comparison: both may present as multiple scattered white patches on the trunk. Distinction between these is important as both have completely different causes and prognosis.

Other differential diagnoses: tinea corporis; post-inflammatory depigmentation; pityriasis alba; idiopathic hypomelanosis; morphoea (p. 92 and Fig. 48.1); lichen sclerosus et atrophicus (p. 96 and Fig. 46.1); piebaldism; naevus anaemicus (Fig. 46.6); occasionally, residual hyperpigmentation may be perceived as abnormal skin and confused with chloasma.

Conclusion and key points: the most useful feature to distinguish between these two conditions is the presence of scaling in untreated pityriasis versicolor but not in vitiligo. This component resolves after treatment but depigmentation may persist for several months and is occasionally permanent. Other useful features to differentiate these disorders are family history, involvement (in vitiligo) of face, hands, or genitalia, and presence of itch in pityriasis versicolor. Wood's light examination of the skin is a useful adjunct in some cases (see Figs 45.2 and 45.4 opposite).

Comparative features		
Disorder	**Pityriasis versicolor**	**Vitiligo**
Age	Young adult (mostly 15–40 yr)	Any
Sex	Either	Female predominance
Family history	May affect partner (unusual)	May be positive for vitiligo, thyroid, or other autoimmune diseases
Sites	Trunk, proximal limbs, neck	Trunk; other common sites are face, hands, genitals
Symptoms	Mild itch, especially after a bath	None, but may burn in sunlight
Signs common to both	Multiple scattered small hypopigmented macules	
Discriminatory signs	Fine scaling is present on untreated lesions, and is best elicited by gentle scraping; note that this resolves after treatment, but that repigmentation does not usually occur until after further sun exposure. The depigmentation may be incomplete, and there may be pink or hyperpigmented lesions on pale skin areas. Lesions may coalesce to form broader patches.	No surface scaling component occurs. Lesions are usually more varied in size, and typically have a margin of slight hyperpigmentation. Follicular repigmentation may produce a spotty mottled appearance. The Koebner reaction may occur (development of lesions at sites of minor injury). Depigmentation of hair may occur in vitiligo but not in pityriasis versicolor.
Associated features	None usually. Dandruff is also due to *Pityrosporum* yeasts but is common and therefore not very helpful diagnostically.	Occasionally halo naevi may be present. Depigmentation of hair can occur at hair-bearing sites including the scalp or eyebrows or eyelashes.
Important tests	Wood's light examination makes the lesions fluoresce and appear paler than the normal skin. Scrape scale for mycology. Consider HIV if pityriasis versicolor is recurrent, resistant to therapy, or the patient is in a high risk group.	Test for other autoimmune disease if there are symptoms.

Further reading:
p. 88, p. 92, p. 96, p. 124.

References
Antoniou C, Katsambas A. Guidelines for the treatment of vitiligo. *Drugs* 1992; **43**:490–8.
Borelli D, Jacobs PH, Nall L. Tinea versicolor: epidemiologic, clinical and therapeutic aspects. *J Am Acad Dermatol* 1991; **25**:300–5.
Laude TA. Approach to dermatologic disorders in black children. *Semin Dermatol* 1995; **14**:15–20.

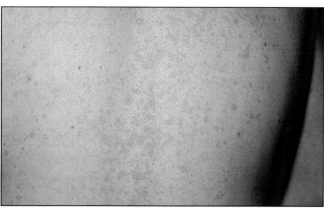

Figure 45.1 *Pityriasis versicolor, showing pigmented lesions on paler normal background skin.*

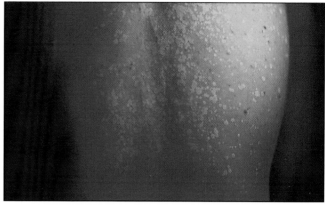

Figure 45.2 *Pityriasis versicolor: Wood's light examination of same patient as in Fig. 45.1. Note that the appearance is now of pale lesions on a darker background.*

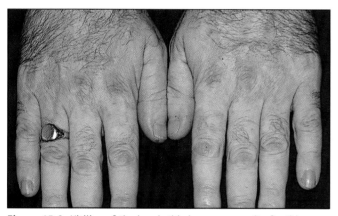

Figure 45.3 *Vitiligo of the hand: this is a common site for this disorder, but rarely affected by pityriasis versicolor.*

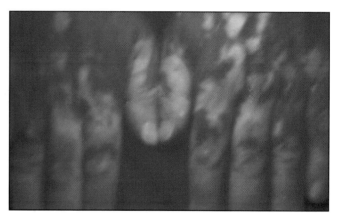

Figure 45.4 *Vitiligo: Wood's light examination of hands (same patient as in Fig. 45.4). In this case, note that the colour difference is accentuated rather than reversed, due to pigment loss.*

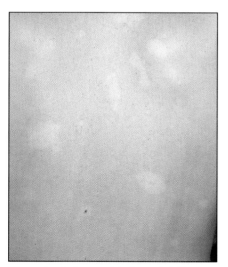

Figure 45.5 *Scattered lesions of vitiligo: the slight marginal hyperpigmentation and the presence of halo naevi differentiate this from pityriasis versicolor.*

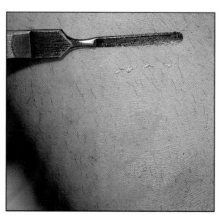

Figure 45.6 *Collecting skin scrapings: this demonstrates the marked scaling in pityriasis versicolor.*

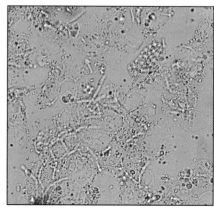

Figure 45.7 *Microscopy of skin scrapings in pityriasis versicolor: this shows the characteristic pattern of yeast spores and hyphae ('bunches of grapes', or 'meatballs and spaghetti').*

46 Lichen sclerosus et atrophicus v. morphoea

Common presenting feature: both disorders may present as either a solitary patch, or as a few, depigmented patches.

Rationale for comparison: these conditions are often confused, particularly when they occur on the trunk. However, they have different treatments and prognoses.

Other differential diagnoses: vitiligo; tinea corporis; pityriasis versicolor (p. 90); post-inflammatory depigmentation; subacute cutaneous lupus erythematosus; granuloma annulare; sarcoidosis; naevus anaemicus.

Conclusion and key points: Lichen sclerosus et atrophicus (LSA) and morphoea are potentially confused if palpation is not a routine part of skin examination: the best distinction is the sclerotic feel of morphoea compared with the atrophic skin texture in LSA. Other distinguishing signs are the purplish border of active morphoea which is not a feature of LSA, the more geographical margin of LSA, and the loss of follicles in morphoea compared with follicular prominence in LSA. Vitiligo, particularly if there are just a few large lesions with marginal hyperpigmentation ('trichrome appearance'), may also cause diagnostic confusion but has normal skin texture.

Comparative features		
Disorder	**Lichen sclerosus et atrophicus (LSA)**	**Morphoea**
Age	Most extragenital LSA occurs in patients aged >40 yr	Any
Sex	Female predominance	Either
Family history	May be positive for autoimmune diseases, e.g. thyroid	Non-specific
Sites	Commonest extragenital site is the trunk	Mainly trunk
Symptoms	May itch	None; itch in early lesions; awareness of sclerosis
Signs common to both	Localized depigmented patches, usually solitary or few in number	
Discriminatory signs	Lesions have an irregular or geographical border, follicular prominence, wrinkled appearance due to atrophy, and ivory or porcelain-white colour. Multiple smaller lesions may coalesce. The Koebner reaction may occur and may explain the relatively high incidence of lesions at the waistline or intertriginous areas.	Involved areas feel hard and sclerotic with a waxy surface texture. The border is usually less sharply defined than in LSA, and there is a purplish inflammatory rim around the sclerotic area in early lesions. Follicles are destroyed (which may be manifest as alopecia in hair-bearing areas). Older lesions have a brownish colour.
Associated features	Genital lesions are commonly present (p. 124)	None
Important tests	None routinely required but investigate if any symptoms of other autoimmune diseases	Localized morphoea is a disorder different from systemic sclerosis, but extensive truncal sclerosis can occur in either generalized morphoea or in systemic sclerosis and such cases require further investigation. See also p.44.

Further reading:
p. 44, p. 90, p. 96, p. 124.

References
Fujiwara H, *et al.* Detection of *Borrelia burgdorferi* DNA (*B. garnii* or *B. afzelii*) in morphoea and lichen sclerosus et atrophicus tissues of German and Japanese but not of US patients. *Arch Dermatol* 1997; **133**:41–4.
Greenberg AS, Falanga V. Localized cutaneous sclerosis. In: Sontheimer RD, Provost TT (eds). *Cutaneous manifestations of rheumatic diseases*. Williams & Wilkins, Baltimore, 1996:177–232.

Wallace HJ. Lichen sclerosus et atrophicus. *Trans Rep St John's Hosp Dermatol Soc* 1971; **57**:9–30.
Katugampola GA, Lanigan SW. The clinical spectrum of naevus anaemicus and its association with port wine stains. *Br J Dermatol* 1996; **134**:292–5.
Meffert JJ, Davis BM, Grinwood RE. Lichen sclerosus. *J Am Acad Dermatol* 1995; **32**:393–416.

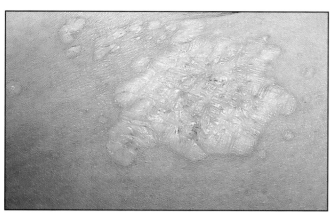

Figure 46.1 *Lichen sclerosus et atrophicus demonstrating follicular prominence and skin atrophy (see also Fig. 15.5).*

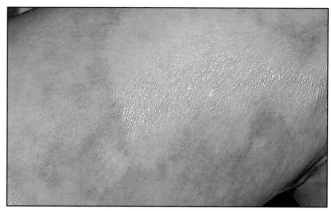

Figure 46.2 *Morphoea, showing a firm, smooth, waxy plaque with violaceous margin.*

Figure 46.3 *Morphoea, similar to that in Fig. 46.2, but with a more active inflammatory margin.*

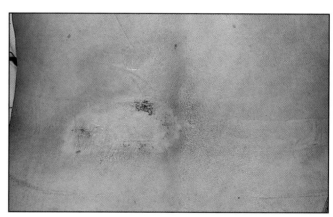

Figure 46.4 *Morphoea and lichen sclerosus et atrophicus: these disorders do appear to occur together in a small proportion of patients and may cause particular diagnostic difficulties. The purpuric component is common in lichen sclerosus et atrophicus due to poor collagen around superficial dermal blood vessels.*

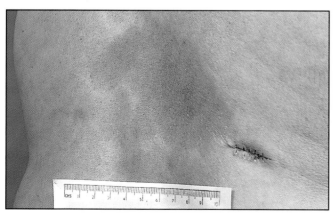

Figure 46.5 *Atrophoderma of Pasini and Pierini: there is typical depressed pigmented skin.*

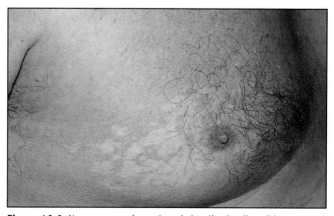

Figure 46.6 *Naevus anaemicus: there is localized pallor with no palpable textural change or thickening, no scaling, and a more geographical outline than in morphoea, lichen sclerosus et atrophicus, or vitiligo. Unlike vitiligo, this lesion disappears under Wood's light.*

47 Polymorphic eruption of pregnancy v. pemphigoid gestationis

Common presenting feature: both disorders cause an intensely itchy dermatosis in pregnancy, characterized by urticated papules and plaques, often with vesicles.

Rationale for comparison: these two eruptions are unique to pregnancy but differ in severity, intensity of treatment required, and prognosis for subsequent pregnancies.

Other differential diagnoses: other pregnancy eruptions (e.g. pruritic folliculitis of pregnancy); eruptions not specific to pregnancy (e.g. scabies, erythema multiforme, drug or viral eruption, contact dermatitis, chickenpox, urticaria, lupus erythematosus).

Conclusion and key points: polymorphic eruption of pregnancy (PEP), which is also known as pruritic urticarial papules and plaques of pregnancy (PUPPP) is much commoner than pemphigoid gestationis (previously called herpes gestationis). PEP starts in the striae, usually in the last few weeks of pregnancy, spares the periumbilical region in 90% of cases, and resolves within a few days of delivery. Pemphigoid gestationis can start at any stage of pregnancy, involves the periumbilical region in 90% of cases, and typically worsens at delivery. Unlike PEP, pemphigoid gestationis may persist for several months after delivery, or may relapse in relation to menstruation or oral contraceptives. It frequently recurs in subsequent pregnancies, whereas PEP is more common in first pregnancies or those with multiple fetuses and does not usually recur in subsequent singleton pregnancies.

Comparative features		
Disorder	**Polymorphic eruption of pregnancy (PEP)**	**Pemphigoid gestationis**
Age and sex	Pregnant female, typically first pregnancy	Pregnant female, any pregnancy
Family history	Non-specific	
Sites	Affects abdomen, thighs, and occasionally distal limbs. The rash usually starts in striae in the last month of pregnancy. The umbilical area is spared in 90% of cases.	Starts on abdomen, initial lesions are periumbilical in 90% of cases, but the rash may affect any body site at any stage of pregnancy (including the post-partum period).
Symptoms	Severe itch	
Signs common to both	Erythematous urticated papules and plaques; vesicles	
Discriminatory signs	Localization to striae. Vesicles are present in 40% of cases but remain small. The rash and itch rapidly regress after delivery.	Periumbilical involvement is typical and annular lesions are more common than in PEP. Vesicles rapidly progress to larger bullae. Exacerbation at the time of delivery is common.
Associated features	None. In particular, the baby is unaffected.	Neonatal involvement may occur due to transplacental transfer of immunoglobulin, causes urticarial lesions and sometimes bullae; these are usually mild and resolve spontaneously.
Important tests	Biopsy with direct immunofluorescence will distinguish between these two disorders	
Prognosis and recurrence	Common (1/250 pregnancies). PEP is typically a disorder of first or multiple pregnancies, especially if there is large weight gain. It resolves rapidly and usually does not recur in subsequent pregnancies.	Rare (1/25 000 pregnancies). This disorder may be severe and require systemic therapy; since introduction of systemic steroids, most studies have not reported increased foetal mortality or morbidity apart from transient rash and some degree of placental insufficiency (slight increase in prematurity and small-for-dates babies). The eruption typically recurs in subsequent pregnancies with the same partner.

Further reading:
pp. 112–116, p. 142.

References
Holmes RC, Black MM. The specific dermatoses of pregnancy: a reappraisal with specific emphasis on a proposed simplified clinical classification. *Clin Exp Dermatol* 1982; **7**:65–73.
Ibbotson SH, Lawrence CM. An uninvolved pregnancy in a patient after a previous episode of herpes gestationis. *Arch Dermatol* 1995; **131**:1091.

Lawley TS, Hertz KC, Wade TR. Pruritic urticarial papules and plaques of pregnancy. *J Am Med Assoc* 1979; **241**:1696–9.
Shornik JK. Pemphigoid (herpes) gestationis. In: Black MM, McKay M, Braude P (eds). *Color atlas and text of obstetric and gynecologic dermatology*. Mosby–Wolfe, London, 1995:29–36.

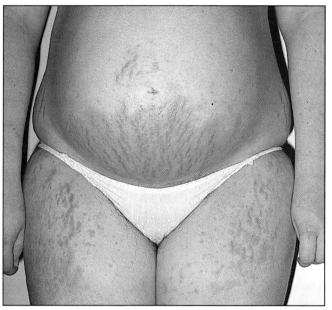

Figure 47.1 *Polymorphic eruption of pregnancy, showing typical distribution on lower abdomen and proximal thighs, with predilection for striae.*

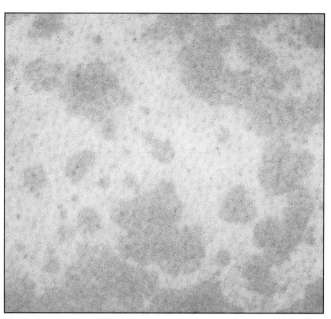

Figure 47.2 *Polymorphic eruption of pregnancy, showing more annular 'urticated' lesions.*

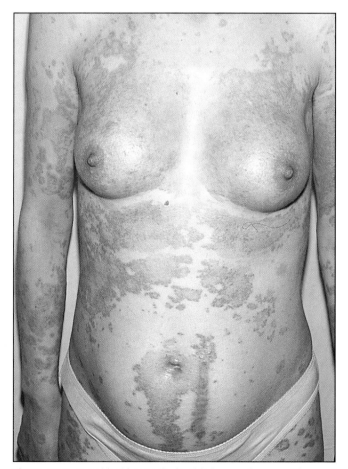

Figure 47.3 *Pemphigoid gestationis: this is a much more widespread eruption, with umbilical involvement.*

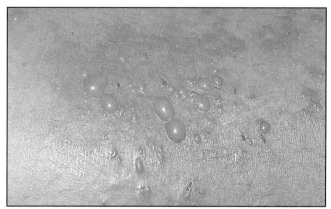

Figure 47.4 *Pemphigoid gestationis, showing tense unilocular blisters, morphologically similar to those in bullous pemphigoid.*

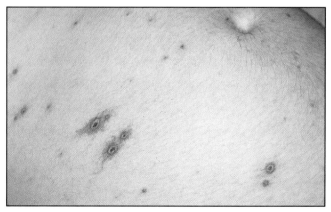

Figure 47.5 *Chickenpox in pregnancy: this causes blisters but a less extensive background eruption. Note that there is a risk of fetal malformations, particularly during gestational weeks 8–22.*

48 Morphoea v. fungal infection (tinea corporis)

Common presenting feature: both conditions may present as relatively asymptomatic discoloured plaque(s), with a distinct border.

Rationale for comparison: many patients with morphoea are initially treated for a fungal infection because both disorders have a distinct inflammatory edge creating an annular shape, and both have central discoloration. However, the physical signs are characteristic and the two disorders can be readily differentiated.

Other differential diagnoses: lichen sclerosus et atrophicus (p. 92); granuloma annulare (p. 72); atrophoderma of Pasini and Pierini; eczemas; parapsoriasis (p. 82); vitiligo (p. 90); lichen planus.

Conclusion and key points: these disorders are often confused because both have an active edge and central discoloration, but they can in fact be readily differentiated. The critical physical sign is the presence or absence of scaling. The skin in tinea corporis is of normal thickness but diffusely scaly, particularly at the advancing margin, while the skin in morphoea is smooth, firm, and waxy. Morphoea has a smoother and generally more rounded border than the enlarging rings of tinea corporis, which often have an irregular shape. The colour of the affected lesion is usually white (or later brownish) in morphoea but greyish in tinea corporis, and the active inflammatory border in morphoea is purplish or violaceous.

Comparative features		
Disorder	**Morphoea**	**Fungal infection (tinea corporis)**
Age	Any, mostly teens and early adult years	
Sex	Either	
Family history	Non-specific	
Sites	Mainly trunk or proximal limbs	Any. Confusion with morphoea is most likely when lesions occur on the trunk.
Symptoms	None; awareness of sclerotic skin	None, itch
Signs common to both	One or few discrete discoloured areas with active border	
Discriminatory signs	Smooth, firm, waxy non-scaling surface. New lesions have a broad purplish-coloured zone of inflammation around them. The centre of lesions is palpably sclerotic and initially white in colour, but may become brown later.	Presence of scaling, particularly at the narrow and slightly irregular advancing edge, is typical but may be altered by topical treatment. The colour is greyish in the centre of lesions. Tinea corporis is typically asymmetrical.
Associated features	None	May be fungal infection at other sites (especially toewebs or nails, scalp in children)
Important tests	Biopsy may be required to support the diagnosis.	Skin scrapings for mycology
Treatment	Usually strong topical corticosteroid	Topical, or occasionally systemic (if multiple lesions or immunosuppressed patient) antifungal agents. Note that topical corticosteroid treatment will initially reduce inflammation and mask the diagnosis (tinea incognito [Figs 55.1–55.5]), but may cause pustular lesions or concentric rings of spreading fungal infection.

Further reading:
p. 82, p. 90, p. 92, p. 110, p. 124.

References

Curtis AC, Jansen TG. The prognosis of localized scleroderma. *Arch Dermatol* 1958; **78**:749–57.

Dabski K, Winkelmann RK. Generalised granuloma annulare: clinical and laboratory findings in 100 patients. *J Am Acad Dermatol* 1989; **20**:39–47.

Hoesly JM, Mertz LE, Winkelmann RK. Localized scleroderma (morphoea) and antibody to *Borrelia burgdorferi*. *J Am Acad Dermatol* 1987; **17**:455–8.

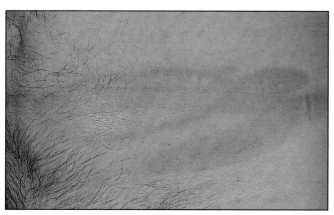

Figure 48.1 *Morphoea, showing shiny, slightly brownish-coloured, plaques with violaceous border (see also p. 92 for further illustrations).*

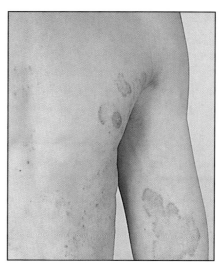

Figure 48.2
Tinea corporis due to Trichophyton verrucosum *from cattle: note the annular shape and active but irregularly shaped borders. This pattern is due to holding the heads of cows while de-horning or administering a drench.*

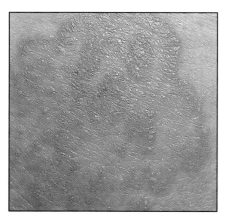

Figure 48.3 *Tinea corporis: the active red border is clearly part of the lesion, rather than a halo around it. Note the presence of scaling.*

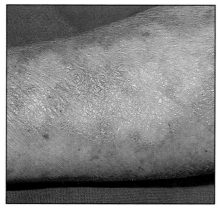

Figure 48.4 *Subacute cutaneous lupus erythematosus: this is a photosensitive pattern of lumpus which resembles tinea, as it is often annular and typically has a scaling component. It also typically has a greyish central colour because the maximal inflammation is at the dermoepidermal junction, causing disruption of pigment and damage to melanocytes.*

Figure 48.5 *Necrobiosis lipoidica demonstrating central atrophic skin and more active inflammatory border. This may be confused with morphoea due to the skin textural abnormality, or with tinea corporis due to the active border.*

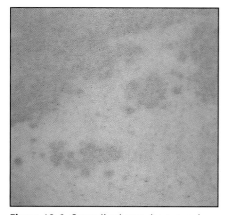

Figure 48.6 *Generalized granuloma annulare: this is a relatively uncommon form of granuloma annulare (1–2% of cases). It often forms rather poorly demarcated plaques with a more prominent papular border, and is particularly confused with tinea corporis.*

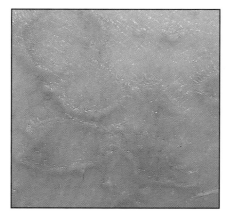

Figure 48.7 *Lichen planus: lesions may be strikingly annular and are typically violaceous.*

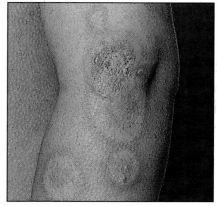

Figure 48.8 *Post-inflammatory hyperpigmentation following erythema multiforme: again, the annular morphology causes confusion with tinea corporis.*

49 Paget's disease v. eczema of nipples

Common presenting feature: a scaly erythematous eruption around the nipple.

Rationale for comparison: Paget's disease is caused by an underlying breast carcinoma and must be diagnosed at an early stage to allow optimal treatment. Conversely, diagnosis of eczema allows reassurance and precludes the need for surgery.

Other differential diagnoses: psoriasis; scabies; seborrhoeic keratosis; parapsoriasis; tinea; jogger's nipple; hyperkeratosis of nipples; Bowen's disease; basal cell carcinoma.

Conclusion and key points: nipple eczema is relatively common. It is sufficiently common in atopic dermatitis to be used as a diagnostic criterion. Nipple eczema is characteristically bilateral, though one side may be more severely affected. By contrast, Paget's disease is unilateral.

Comparative features		
Disorder	**Paget's disease of breast**	**Eczema of nipples**
Age	Mostly >40 yr	Mostly young adult
Sex	Virtually all patients are female, but either condition can occasionally occur in men.	
Family history	Non-specific	May be atopic
Sites	Nipple and adjacent areola: unilateral	Nipple and adjacent areola: bilateral
Symptoms	None, itch	Usually severe itch
Signs common to both	Scaly erythematous eruption of nipple and adjacent areola	
Discriminatory signs	Unilateral, progressive, raised red lesion with a well defined edge. There may be a palpable neoplasm but Paget's disease is often due to a small superficial and impalpable intraductal carcinoma. Nipple discharge may occur in some cases.	Bilateral but not necessarily symmetrical in degree. Typically moist and crusted with fissuring. May be variable in intensity, and shows some response to therapy (although it is often relatively refractory).
Associated features	Underlying neoplasm	May be other atopic features, or history of reactions to cheap metals
Important tests	Biopsy for histology (special stains will demonstrate characteristic glycogen content of the infiltrating cells). Mammography, surgery	Biopsy if any doubt. Bacteriology swab, as chronic eczema at this site is almost inevitably associated with staphylococcal infection. Patch testing

Further reading:
p. 102, p. 106.

References

MacKie RM. *Skin cancer*, 2nd edn. Martin Dunitz, London, 1996:96–9.

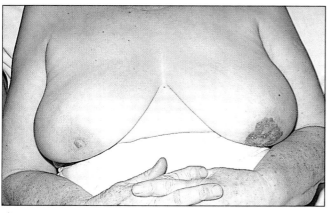

Figure 49.1 *Paget's disease of nipple: this is a unilateral disorder.*

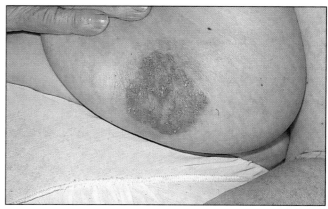

Figure 49.2 *Paget's disease of nipple (close-up).*

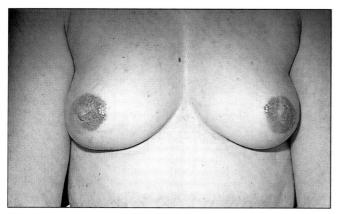

Figure 49.3 *Nipple eczema is bilateral: this patient had a positive patch test to nickel, which is relatively common in patients with this problem, though the relevance is obscure in most cases.*

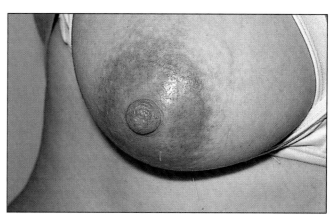

Figure 49.4 *Psoriasis of nipple, occurring as a Koebner reaction due to breast-feeding.*

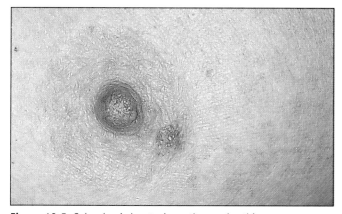

Figure 49.5 *Seborrhoeic keratosis on the areola: this may cause concern about Paget's disease.*

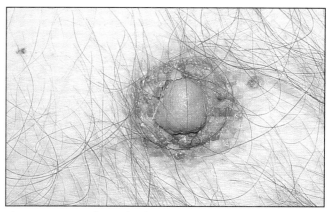

Figure 49.6 *Hyperkeratosis of nipple: this is a disorder which mainly affects elderly men.*

50 Cholinergic urticaria v. flushing

Common presenting feature: episodic, often stress-related, upper truncal erythema.

Rationale for comparison: the causes, investigation, and management of these conditions are different.

Other differential diagnoses: other forms of urticaria or dermographism; vascular anomalies.

Conclusion and key points: flushing is not associated with itch, rarely has any significant underlying cause, and neither disorder requires nor responds well to treatment.

The presence of an underlying systemic cause should be considered if there is associated hypotension, hypertension, tachycardia, respiratory or gastrointestinal symptoms, or if there is fixed erythema in a flush distribution. Cholinergic urticaria is often triggered by a range of stimuli, such as stress, exercise and hot conditions (some of which may also trigger flushing); it is differentiated by the presence of small papules with a surrounding vascular flare. These tiny weals are transient and may be prevented by taking oral antihistamines, though not all individuals respond well.

Comparative features		
Disorder	**Cholinergic urticaria**	**Flushing**
Age	Young adult	Any, often young adult
Sex	Mainly male	Mainly female
Family history	Non-specific	
Sites	Trunk, arms	Upper trunk, upper arms, face
Symptoms	Itch	None, or awareness of feeling hot or flushed
Signs common to both	Transient patchy erythema affecting the upper trunk; may be provoked by stress or emotional stimuli	
Discriminatory signs	Lesions are papular and mainly discrete, may have a small central weal and have a surrounding vascular flare.	Confluent areas of erythema, with irregular geographical margins. Itch and weals do not occur.
Associated features	May be triggered by emotion or stress but typically occurs in a hot environment or during exercise, which acts as a stimulus to sweating. Other physical urticarias may occur in the same individual, e.g. dermographism.	Mainly emotion or stress triggered but may be other specific triggers (alcohol, solvents, medications). Systemic symptoms (bronchoconstriction, hypotension) suggest a metabolic cause. Fixed telangiectasia suggests carcinoid syndrome.
Important tests	None are routinely required but lesions can be provoked by a warm bath (41–42°C for 10–15 minutes) or by exercise (sufficient to provoke sweating) to confirm the diagnosis. A therapeutic response to oral antihistamines is also useful support but not all patients respond well.	None unless there are associated systemic symptoms (consider hormone-producing tumours, e.g. carcinoid, phaeochromocytoma)

Further reading:
p. 112.

References
Cox NH, Mustchin CP. Prolonged spontaneous and alcohol-induced flushing due to the solvent dimethylformamide. *Contact Dermatitis* 1991; **24**:69–70.
Harada S, Agarwal DP, Goedda HW. Aldehyde dehydrogenase deficiency as a cause of facial flushing reaction to alcohol in Japanese. *Lancet* 1981; **ii**:982.

Janmohammed S, Bloom SR. Carcinoid tumours. *Postgrad Med J* 1997; **73**:207–14.
Wilkin JK. The red face: flushing disorders. *Clin Dermatol* 1993; **11**:211–23.
Wilkin JK. Why is flushing limited to a mostly facial cutaneous distribution? *J Am Acad Dermatol* 1988; **19**:309–13.
Zuberbier T, *et al.* Prevalence of cholinergic urticaria in young adults. *J Am Acad Dermatol* 1994; **31**:978–81.

Some causes of flushing	
Generalized	Emotional, menopausal, thermal Drugs – alcohol (alone, or with griseofulvin, metronidazole, or chlorpropamide), vasodilators, food additives, inhaled solvents (trichloroethylene, dimethyl formamide, N-butylraldoxine) Pathological – mastocytosis, carcinoid, phaeochromocytoma, peptide-secreting tumours
Localized	Dermographism Response to skin injury Rosacea Erythromelalgia

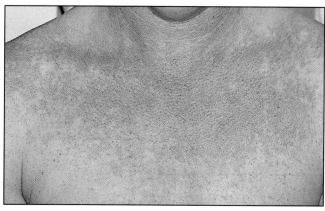

Figure 50.1 *Physiological flushing, showing typical upper truncal distribution.*

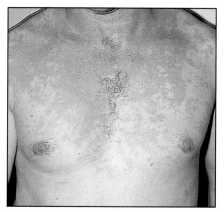

Figure 50.2 *Flushing due to a solvent (dimethylformamide): this is diagnosed from the history as the distribution is similar to that of physiological flushing.*

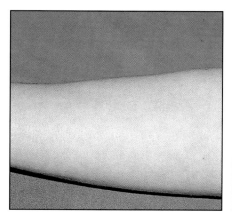

Figures 50.3 and 50.4 *Cholinergic urticaria: provocation of lesions by exercise.*

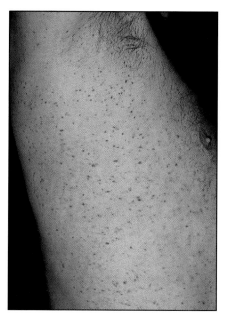

Figure 50.5
Urticaria pigmentosa: patients with scattered tiny lesions may have small itchy weals similar to those of cholinergic urticaria. They are, however, fixed in position, and become red after rubbing them—this response, known as Darier's sign, occurs because mechanical degranulation of mast cells allows release of histamine and other inflammatory mediators.

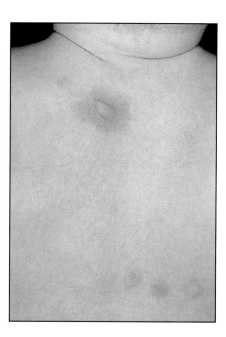

Figure 50.6
Urticaria pigmentosa, showing a more typical pattern of fewer and larger fixed brown plaques, with prominent Darier's sign.

51 Psoriasis v. discoid eczema (nummular dermatitis)

Common presenting feature: both disorders cause a rash which typically consists of scattered small plaques.

Rationale for comparison: these two disorders are often confused unless there is a preceding history of more localized psoriasis. There is a wider range of treatment options for psoriasis, but some of the agents used may potentially worsen discoid eczema.

Other differential diagnoses: tinea corporis (p. 110 and Fig. 48.2); pityriasis versicolor (p. 90); lichen planus; parapsoriasis or mycosis fungoides (p. 82, p. 84); drug eruption (e.g. methyl dopa); Bowen's disease; superficial basal cell carcinomas (p. 86).

Conclusion and key points: the key difference is the degree of itch, which is usually very prominent in discoid eczema but absent or less severe in psoriasis. Useful distinguishing physical signs are the body site distribution (discoid eczema mainly affects the limbs, but not specifically the extensor aspects of elbows and knees, which are typical sites for psoriasis), and close-up morphology (psoriasis has silvery scaling whereas active discoid eczema is moist or crusted). Therapies such as dithranol (anthralin) and calcipotriol are useful agents for treating psoriasis but will aggravate discoid eczema.

Comparative features		
Disorder	**Plaque psoriasis**	**Discoid eczema**
Age	Any. The peak age of onset is the 2nd to 3rd decade	Any. The peak age of onset is in 6th decade
Sex	Either	
Family history	Often positive	Non-specific. Discoid lesions can occur in atopics, in which case there may be a positive family history.
Sites	Any. In extensive psoriasis, it is usual that the distribution of lesions will include the characteristic sites for more limited disease, such as the extensor aspect of knees and elbows, scalp (especially forehead scalp margin and above ears), sacrum or gluteal area.	Any, but predominantly limbs
Symptoms	None, itch	Usually very marked itch. Lesions may be tender or painful because secondary infection is common.
Signs common to both	Scattered, discrete, sharply demarcated, erythematous plaques	
Discriminatory signs	Usually silvery-white surface scale, with typical site distribution, and there may be a Koebner reaction (Fig. 40.2).	Discoid eczema is more exudative, therefore the surface is moist or crusted in the active phase. Fine scale is present in the resolving phase.
Associated features	May be associated arthropathy, or nail signs (p. 174)	None
Important tests	None	Lesions are often secondarily infected, therefore send bacteriology swabs to guide antibiotic treatment.

Further reading:
p. 2, pp. 58–64, pp. 80–84, p. 118, p. 134, p. 150, p. 174.

References
Calnan CD, Meara RH. Discoid eczema—dry type. *Trans St John's Hosp Dermatol Soc* 1956; **37**:26–8.

Cowan MA. Nummular eczema—a review, follow-up and analysis of 325 cases. *Acta Dermatovenereol* 1961; **41**:453–60.
Church R. Eczema provoked by methyldopa. *Br J Dermatol* 1974; **91**:373–8.

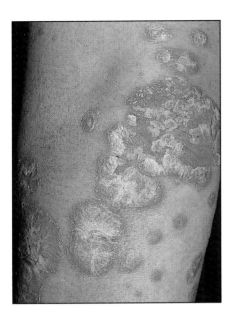

Figure 51.1 *Typical plaque psoriasis, showing a well-defined border and silvery scale.*

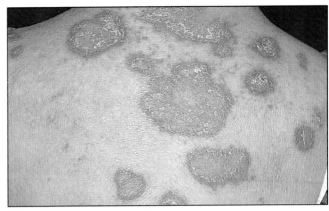

Figure 51.2 *Truncal plaques of psoriasis, with lesions of a more uniform size.*

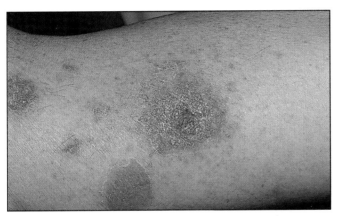

Figure 51.3 *Typical discoid eczema: the lesions are weeping, crusted, and poorly demarcated.*

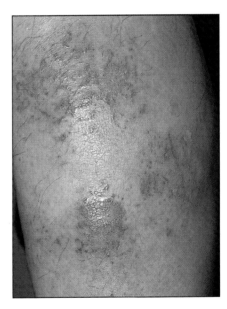

Figure 51.4 *Discoid eczema: there are less acute lesions, with poorly demarcated borders.*

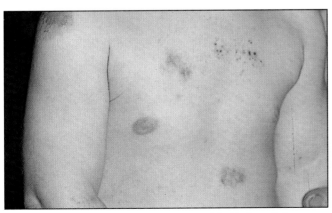

Figure 51.5 *Discoid lesions in an atopic child: this is an infrequent pattern in this age-group.*

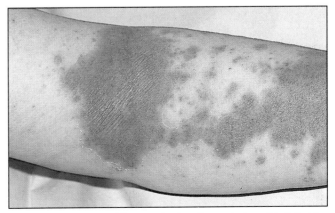

Figure 51.6 *Eczema: this was mistaken for psoriasis and irritated by topical treatment for this diagnosis.*

Common presenting feature: these two disorders may both cause a generalized, often maculopapular, rash.

Rationale for comparison: because an antibiotic may be prescribed during the early stages of a febrile illness, the occurrence of rash a few days later is generally assumed to represent antibiotic allergy rather than a viral exanthem. If an assumption of antibiotic allergy is erroneous, it may incorrectly preclude use of the antibiotic for subsequent infections.

Other differential diagnoses: urticaria (p. 112); guttate psoriasis (p. 80); scabies (p. 106); streptococcal infections; secondary syphilis; other types of eruption which may be due to either drugs or infection (e.g. erythema multiforme, see p. 112).

Conclusion and key points: there is no simple method to distinguish between these diagnoses. A convincing history of upper respiratory tract or influenza-like infection favours the diagnosis of a viral exanthem, especially if supported by a rising antibody titre to a relevant virus on paired serology samples. Rapid resolution after stopping a suspect drug favours this as a cause but may occur due to spontaneous resolution of a viral exanthem. Distinguishing between different drug causes in patients taking multiple agents is largely on the basis of timing, type and frequency of rash anticipated with the different drugs. Note three important guiding points: 1. Most drug eruptions commence 3–10 days after starting the drug. In the case of antibiotics prescribed as a short course, a drug eruption may therefore begin after a course of treatment, or may worsen for a few days after stopping the relevant drug. Such a history is often incorrectly thought to exonerate the suspect agent. 2. Some penicillins, particularly ampicillin and derivatives, are more likely to cause a rash when used in patients with a viral infection (particularly infectious mononucleosis) compared with the frequency of rash when used to treat bacterial infections. 3. Most drug reactions continue to worsen unless the drug is stopped, but viral exanthems will all fade and disappear.

Comparative features		
Disorder	**Drug eruption**	**Viral exanthem**
Age	Any, mainly adults	Any, mainly children
Sex	Either	
Family history	Non-specific	There may be other family members with exanthem or symptoms of infection
Sites	Generalized, usually mainly truncal	Generalized; some start as facial rash, e.g. measles
Symptoms	None/itch	
Signs common to both	Both cause a generalized maculopapular eruption which may heal with a fine desquamating phase. Either may preferentially spare pressure areas under clothing. Lymphadenopathy, malaise, fever, conjunctivitis, and elevated levels of hepatic transaminases may occur in either case.	
Discriminatory signs	None specific. Residual hyperpigmentation favours a drug-induced cause.	None, although some may have a characteristic pattern (e.g. Gianotti–Crosti syndrome, Fig. 40.5), or may fulfil a set of diagnostic criteria (e.g. Kawasaki disease). There may be useful mucous membrane changes, e.g. Koplik's spots in measles, palatal petechiae and enlarged tonsils in infectious mononucleosis.
Associated features	Usually the suspect drug was started within 10 days prior to rash. Presence of eosinophilia favours a drug-induced exanthematous rash.	There are usually preceding upper respiratory or influenza-like symptoms. Photophobia or respiratory symptoms favour an infective cause.
Important tests	Stop drug; rechallenge if it is important to know with certainty which drug caused the reaction, and provided the reaction was not severe.	Throat swab/other direct bacteriology. Serology for viral titres, stool cultures etc. if clinically indicated. HIV or syphilis serology in some cases
Evolution	Most eruptions settle within a few days of stopping the suspect drug, but some start after the course of medication is completed.	Most eruptions settle within a week or two, but may persist for several weeks in some types of exanthem.

Drugs which commonly cause exanthematous eruptions	
Antibiotics	Penicillins/cephalosporins, sulphonamides
Anticonvulsants	Carbamazepine, phenytoin
Rheumatology	NSAIDs, gold, allopurinol

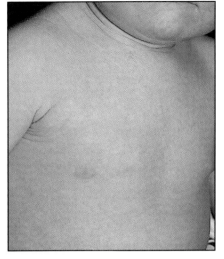

Figure 52.1
Exanthem in a child, showing a common and non-specific pattern.

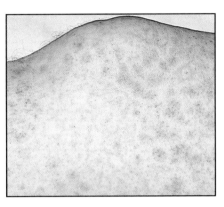

Figure 52.2
Generalized rash due to amoxicillin (shown here on the knee). The drug was prescribed for a patient who was later demonstrated to have infectious mononucleosis.

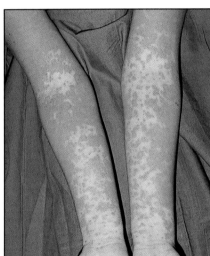

Figure 52.3
Extensive, 'urticated' eruption due to phenytoin. Anticonvulsants are relatively frequent causes of a drug eruption.

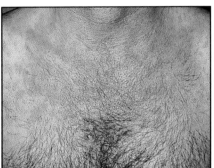

Figure 52.4
Maculopapular rash in a man with preceding respiratory symptoms. No cause was identified, but a viral exanthem was likely as he had not taken any medication.

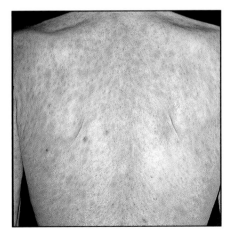

Figure 52.5
Extensive rash with a pattern suggestive of pityriasis rosea (rather oval lesions following dermatomal orientation on the back, the so-called fir-tree pattern). Several patients with a similar rash were seen over a period of a few months, but no causative virus was identified.

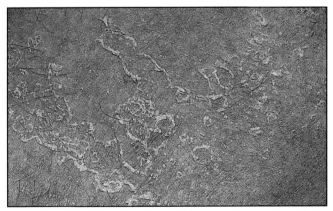

Figure 52.6 *Loose scaling in the resolving phase of a drug reaction.*

Further reading:
p. 80, p. 106, p. 112.

References
Anonymous. Ampicillin rashes. *BMJ* 1975; **ii**:7089.
Goodyear HM, *et al*. Acute infectious erythemas in children: a clinico-microbiological study. *Br J Dermatol* 1991; **124**:433–8.

Bialecki C, Feder HM, Grant–Kels JM. The six classic childhood exanthems. *J Am Acad Dermatol* 1989; **21**:891–903.
Bork K. *Cutaneous side-effects of drugs.* WB Saunders, Philadelphia, 1988.

Atopic eczema v. scabies

Common presenting feature: both disorders cause an itch with an eczematous rash.

Rationale for comparison: recognition of scabies is important as it is readily curable.

Other differential diagnoses: other forms of eczema; urticaria (weals are frequent in scabies); pemphigoid (p. 114, p. 142); impetigo; excoriations in generalized pruritus.

Conclusion and key points: vigilance is the key factor in diagnosis of scabies. The presence of preceding atopic eczema does not preclude the diagnosis of scabies, but does raise other possibilities (particularly secondary

bacterial or herpetic infection in an atopic). Lesions of fingerwebs, wrists, breasts, or penis/scrotum are common in scabies.

Apparent 'eczema' that starts for the first time after infancy, or an eczematous rash starting at about the same time in several family members, both give rise to the suspicion of scabies. Note that itch may take up to 3 months to develop after initial infestation, so the family history may well be negative in the earliest stages. Burrows are diagnostic but may be difficult to differentiate from small scratches; extracting a scabies mite and demonstrating it to the patient down the microscope is useful as there is no subsequent doubt about the diagnosis in either the medical records or in the mind of a sceptical patient.

Comparative features		
Disorder	**Atopic eczema**	**Scabies**
Age	Any. Usually starts in first six months of life, and severity decreases in older children	Any. Particularly common in school children and young adults
Sex	Either	
Family history	Often positive but often historical	Often positive. Concurrent or recent onset of itch is commonly present amongst household, family, school or sexual contacts
Sites	Infant: generalized Older child: antecubital, popliteal, wrists, ankles	Infant: soles of feet plus generalized papules Older child: Hands, generalized, genital Post-pubertal: also affects breasts and penis
Symptoms	Itch, may be severe but has usually been present to some extent for a more prolonged period	Profound itch, especially nocturnal; of recent onset
Signs common to both	Eczematous rash +/- excoriation, crusting, secondary infection	
Discriminatory signs	Flexural distribution is usually present in conjunction with a more widespread rash. Lesions are usually patches or thin plaques and may be lichenified. Eczema of the nipple area is a feature in teenagers/young adults but is more confluent in pattern than the scattered papular periareolar lesions that occur in scabies.	Burrows are pathognomonic, and are best seen on the fingers or borders of the palm. The scattered lesions which occur as a reaction to the infestation are generally papular rather than larger eczematous patches. Scattered weals are common. Penile nodules, or periareolar lesions in women, are strongly indicative. Scabetic nodules occur in disease of longer duration, and particularly affect the penis, scrotum and axillae.
Associated features	Other atopic disorders, e.g. asthma, hayfever. However, beware that these do not preclude a diagnosis of scabies.	Scattered impetigo including the hands is suspicious in an itchy child.
Important tests	None routinely required	Positive identification of a mite (or eggs/faeces) is helpful.
Therapeutic points	Individuals with atopic eczema can also become infested with scabies.	Treat *all* likely family/sexual or same-household contacts

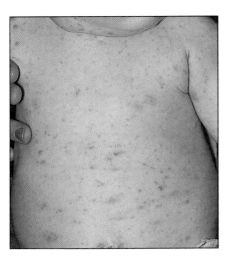

Figure 53.1 *Scabies in an infant. This 'buckshot' pattern of slightly urticarial-appearing lesions is characteristic of the immunological reaction to scabies.*

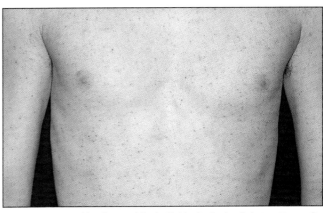

Figure 53.2 *Scabies in an older individual: the buckshot pattern of widespread tiny eczematous lesions triggered by scabies.*

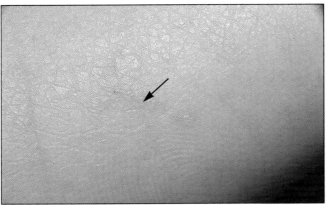

Figure 53.3 *Close-up of scabies burrow: the grey dot at the end of the burrow is the region from which the egg-laying adult female can be extracted.*

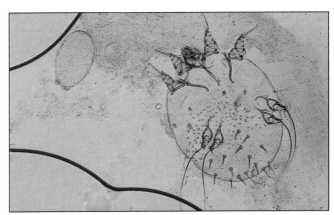

Figure 53.4 *Microscopy of scabies mite and egg.*

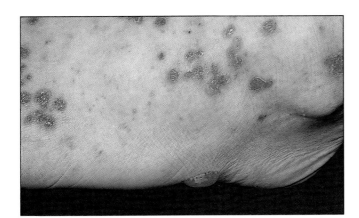

Figure 53.5 *Scabies on the foot of a child: blisters may occur (see also Figs. 33.5, 33.6).*

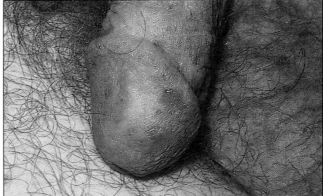

Figure 53.6 *Scabies nodules on the glans penis are a diagnostic feature.*

Further reading:
p. 26, p. 66, p. 98, p. 108, p. 112, p. 114, p. 132, p. 142.

References
Cox NH, Paterson WD. Epidemiology of scabies: the new epidemic. *Lancet* 1991; i:1547–8.
Forsman KE. Pediculosis and scabies. What to look for in patients who are crawling with clues. *Postgrad Med* 1995; **98**:89–100.

Meinking TL, Taplin D. Safety of permethrin vs. lindane for the treatment of scabies. *Arch Dermatol* 1996; **132**:959–62.
Pryzibilla B, Eberlein-Konig B, Rueff F. Practical management of atopic eczema. *Lancet* 1994; **343**:1342–6.

54 Dermatitis herpetiformis v. eczema

Common presenting feature: itchy rash.

Rationale for comparison: specific systemic treatment is required for dermatitis herpetiformis, and evidence of associated malabsorption should be sought.

Other differential diagnoses: scabies; pruritus with localized excoriations; nodular prurigo; urticaria; erythema multiforme; linear IgA disease; pemphigoid.

Conclusion and key points: an itchy rash with vesicles localized to extensor elbows and/or knees, sacrum, upper back, and scalp is strongly suggestive of dermatitis herpetiformis (DH). However, the degree of itch is such that the patient may have scratched early papules or vesicles and may therefore not be aware of the presence of blisters. Skin biopsy with immunofluorescence for IgA deposition is therefore important if the history and distribution of excoriations is suggestive of DH, even if no intact vesicles are visualized. Proof of the diagnosis is important, as DH generally requires life-long therapy which may be both complicated (gluten-free diet) and have significant potential side-effects (dapsone).

Comparative features		
Disorder	**Dermatitis herpetiformis (DH)**	**Eczema**
Age	Any	
Sex	Either	
Family history	Occasionally positive for DH or coeliac disease	Non-specific (may be positive if atopic)
Sites	Extensor elbows/knees, scalp, sacrum/lumbar area, scapular area, ears	Any, but eczematous lesions and excoriations may have a distribution similar to that of DH, especially if pruritus is severe
Symptoms	Itch (severe). Rarely, patients may have symptoms of associated malabsorption (coeliac disease).	Itch, may be severe
Signs common to both	Excoriations, papular or raised red 'urticated' lesions, vesicles	
Discriminatory signs	Vesicles are more likely in DH, but may be excoriated. Haemorrhagic palmar or oral mucosal lesions are uncommon but strongly favour a diagnosis of DH.	The body site distribution of eczemas is more widespread than the relatively specific sites of lesions in DH. Multilocular vesicles and lichenification are eczematous features.
Associated features	Malabsorption due to associated coeliac disease may be a feature, but is usually not symptomatic.	May be other symptoms depending on the cause of eczema, e.g. atopic symptoms such as asthma
Important tests	Skin biopsy; this must include immunofluorescence for IgA deposition. Assess for evidence of malabsorption (biochemical, anti-gliaden antibodies, jejunal biopsy if required).	Elevated serum IgE may be useful to confirm atopic status.
Treatment	Dapsone gives rapid symptomatic improvement but is a potentially toxic drug and requires careful monitoring in the early stage of treatment. Gluten-free diet is effective but much slower to work, and often does not avoid the need for dapsone although it may allow reduction of the dose required. It is less acceptable to patients with DH compared to those with coeliac disease, as most have no gastrointestinal symptoms.	Usually emollients, topical corticosteroids, bandages, antibiotics or antiseptics for secondary infection, oral antihistamines, occasionally other systemic therapies

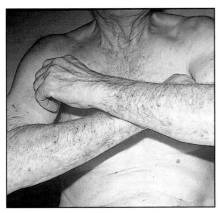

Figure 54.1 *Dermatitis herpetiformis, showing typical distribution on extensor forearms.*

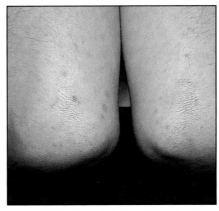

Figure 54.2 *Dermatitis herpetiformis: closer view of typical small papular and excoriated lesions.*

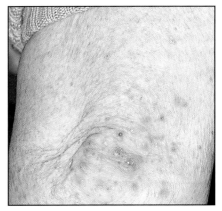

Figure 54.3 *Scabies: papular lesions concentrated at the extensor aspect of the elbow is a relatively frequent pattern. This distribution, and the intense itch, may suggest a diagnosis of dermatitis herpetiformis.*

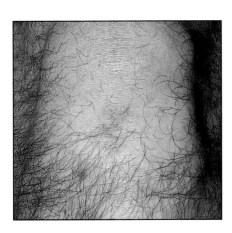

Figure 54.4 *Dermatitis herpetiformis: there are urticated papules and small blisters on the extensor aspect of the knees, another typical site.*

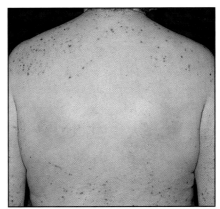

Figure 54.5 *Generalized pruritus with small excoriations limited to accessible sites, (a pattern known as the 'butterfly sign', see also Fig. 57.4). This may be mistaken for DH, as the latter typically affects sacrum and scapulae and is also very itchy.*

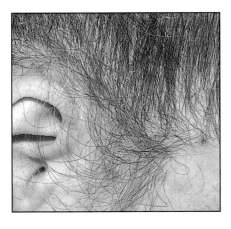

Figure 54.6 *Small vesicles and excoriations in the scalp: this patient actually had linear IgA disease, but the appearance is very similar to dermatitis herpetiformis (DH). The scalp is a very typical but often underestimated site of lesions in DH.*

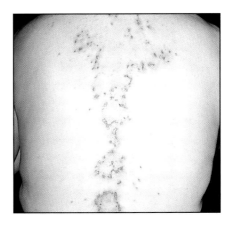

Figure 54.7 *Linear IgA disease. By comparison with DH, the blisters are often larger and have a tendency to coalesce in annular patterns.*

Further reading:
p. 26, p. 74, p. 106, p. 112, p. 114, p.142.

References
Fry L. Dermatitis herpetiformis. In: Wojnarowska F, Briggaman RA (eds). *Management of blistering disorders*. Chapman & Hall, London, 1990; 139–60.

Gordon S, Loewenthal LJA. Chronic eczema as a variant of dermatitis herpetiformis. *Br J Dermatol* 1949; **61**:359–78.
Hall RP. Dermatitis herpetiformis. *J Invest Dermatol* 1992; **99**:873–81.
Leonard JN, Tucker WFG, Fry JS. Increased incidence of malignancy in dermatitis herpetiformis. *BMJ* 1983; **286**:16–18.

Common presenting feature: scaly itchy rash.

Rationale for comparison: there are important therapeutic and prognostic differences between these two disorders. There is a risk of masking and worsening tinea if the problem is inadvertently treated as eczema.

Other differential diagnoses: annular and discoid rashes at various body sites, including psoriasis; lichen planus; subacute cutaneous lupus erythematosus; pityriasis versicolor; erythrasma; parapsoriasis/mycosis fungoides; morphoea; Darier's disease; seborrhoeic dermatitis; granuloma annulare; erythema chronicum migrans (Lyme disease).

Conclusion and key points: the only certain way to determine the presence of a tinea (dermatophyte) infection is to examine scrapings or send them for mycology.

Untreated tinea has fine scaling, and usually has an annular morphology with a red 'active' advancing edge. However, these features may be less obvious if the eruption is partially treated. Antifungal treatment may interfere with viability of fungi and therefore cause false-negative mycology results; if the patient is partially treated but not responding well at the time that the diagnosis of fungal infection is considered, then topical treatment should be stopped for a fortnight in order to obtain valid scrapings for mycology. Topical corticosteroid therapy may mask the fungal infection by reducing inflammation, but the fungus will continue to proliferate. Taking skin scrapings before starting treatment will avoid both of these pitfalls.

Always consider tinea if an apparent eczematous eruption is asymmetrical, and always examine the feet for athlete's foot or tinea of the toenails where any doubt exists, as these are commonly the source of the infection. See also pages 58 and 62.

Comparative features		
Disorder	**Tinea (excluding palms/soles)**	**Eczemas**
Age	Any	
Sex	Either	
Family history	Non-specific	A positive history does not exclude the possibility of tinea.
Sites	Any. Typically asymmetrical (Fig. 31.1) except on the feet	Any. Typically symmetrical unless specific localizing cause, e.g. some contact dermatitis
Symptoms	Itch (usually mild-moderate)	Itch (usually moderate to severe)
Signs common to both	Erythematous scaly patch(es)/plaque(s), may be annular	
Discriminatory signs	The annular ring-like morphology is usually prominent if untreated (Fig. 48.2). There is fine scaling which is accentuated at the periphery (Fig. 48.3); some types of fungi are more inflammatory and may cause pustules or blisters (Fig. 31.2). Fungal infections, other than of the feet, are typically asymmetrical.	Usually symmetrical (Fig. 31.3). Eczemas are typically more itchy, and therefore more excoriated, than tinea. Annular and discoid patterns may occur (p. 102) but patches of eczema have a less distinct margin by comparison with tinea. There may be other eczematous features, eg. vesiculation, lichenification (Fig. 59.3). Look for other features of specific types of eczema, e.g. atopics with annular lesions may have symmetrical flexural eczema.
Associated features	Tinea pedis or tinea unguium (pp. 170–172, p. 176). Fungal infections on the foot are often chronic and the patient may not recognize them as abnormal, therefore make a point of specifically examining the feet even if the patient denies any abnormality.	Eczematous nail changes (p.174)
Important tests	Skin scrapes for mycology. Specific tests to exclude other differential diagnoses may be required (e.g. serology for subacute cutaneous lupus erythematosus, Fig. 48.4).	Patch tests. IgE level is sometimes required to support a diagnosis of atopy.
Comment on treatment	Blind systemic antifungal therapy is rarely justifiable, and may produce side-effects.	Corticosteroid therapy of tinea will mask the clinical signs (tinea incognito).

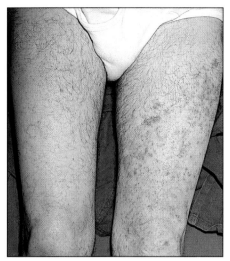
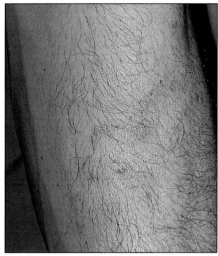
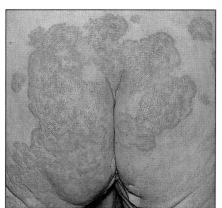
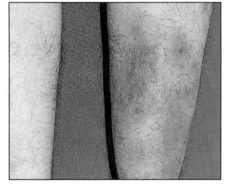
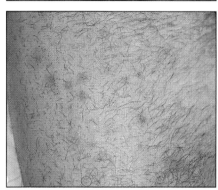

Figures 55.1–55.5 *These are all examples of fungal infection masked by topical corticosteroids, so-called tinea incognito. All show one or more of the following features: asymmetry, accentuation of the eruption at the border, annular morphology, or pustules.*

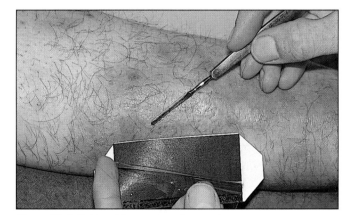

Figure 55.6 *Taking skin scrapings for mycology.*

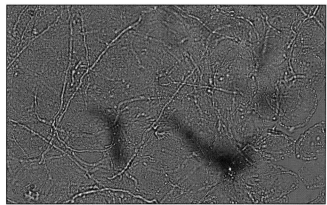

Figure 55.7 *Appearance of fungal hyphae in a potassium hydroxide preparation.*

Further reading:
p. 28, p. 58, p. 62, p. 68, p. 96, p. 118, p. 120,
   p. 132, pp. 170–176.

References
Drake LA, *et al*. Guidelines of care for superficial mycotic infections of the skin: tinea corporis, tinea cruris, tinea facei, tinea manuum and tinea pedis. *J Am Acad Dermatol* 1996; **34**:282–6.

Elewski BE. Cutaneous mycoses in children. *Br J Dermatol* 1996; **134**(Suppl 46):7–11, 37–8.
Terragni L, *et al*. Tinea corporis bullosa. *Mycoses* 1993; **36**:135–7.

Common presenting feature: acute eruption of raised annular lesions.

Rationale for comparison: these conditions are often confused, but have different aetiologies and treatment.

Other differential diagnoses: other patterns of drug eruption; vasculitis; early stage of bullous pemphigoid; fungal infections; Sweet's disease; papular urticaria (p. 142); panniculitis (Fig. 74.7).

Conclusion and key points: erythema multiforme is an eruption with specific histological features, rather than a term which should be used for any eruption of mixed morphology. It can readily be differentiated from urticaria, as the lesions of erythema multiforme are fixed in position, and do not show day-to-day variation as occurs in urticaria. If patients are uncertain about this, the diagnosis can easily be proven by drawing around a lesion and reviewing it the next day. Target lesions have multiple concentric rings, not just a single annular component. Note that patients often confuse weals with blisters, but weals do not burst or leak fluid when pricked. Erythema multiforme may occur as a pattern of drug reaction, but the most frequent trigger is herpes simplex virus infection.

Comparative features		
Disorder	**Erythema multiforme**	**Urticaria**
Age	Any. Herpes simplex is the usual trigger in children and young adults. Drug reactions are a more common cause in older patients.	Any
Sex	Either	
Family history	Negative	May be positive
Sites	Any site. The limbs are more frequently affected than the trunk. Classic 'target' lesions are most frequent on palms. The mucous membranes may be affected (Stevens–Johnson syndrome).	Any. Acute severe urticaria may also be manifest as deeper swelling (angioedema, p. 24) of lips, tongue, or extremities.
Symptoms	None, itch. May be associated fever and malaise	Itch or burning sensation, may be severe
Signs common to both	Discrete, erythematous, annular plaques. Neither has a scaling component (compare tinea, p. 110) although resolving erythema multiforme may scab or crust.	
Discriminatory signs	Multiple concentric 'target' lesions are characteristic but are not required to make the diagnosis, nor are lesions with a target morphology specific to erythema multiforme. The centre of the lesions may be bullous or necrotic. Lesions are fixed, but may enlarge over several days. Residual, sometimes annular, hyperpigmentation may occur.	Lesions vary in number and position over a few hours (<24 hr). In annular lesions, the central skin may be normal, oedematous or occasionally purpuric, but with no epidermal change or blistering. Associated dermographism may occur. Erosive mucosal lesions may occur in erythema multiforme but are not a feature of urticaria.
Associated features	A history of preceding drugs or herpes simplex may be elicited, or there may be residual signs of herpes simplex.	Anaphylaxis, wheeze, intraoral swelling in acute severe cases
Important tests	Often none. Proof of a causative herpes simplex or other infection may require direct swabs, serology etc. Skin biopsy to confirm the diagnosis is advisable in severe or recurrent cases where systemic therapy is considered.	Often none. Test for physical urticarias as indicated by the history. Chronic urticaria justifies investigation, which is usually negative, but does not enter the differential diagnosis of erythema multiforme.

Some causes of erythema multiforme	
Infections	Herpes simplex, orf, *Mycoplasma*, hepatitis, streptococcal
Drugs	Sulphonamides, penicillins, anticonvulsants, NSAIDs, oestrogens
Other	Lupus erythematosus, inflammatory bowel disease, neoplasia, idiopathic

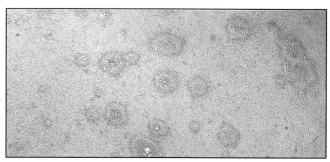

Figure 56.1 *Erythema multiforme, with 'target' lesions on the trunk.*

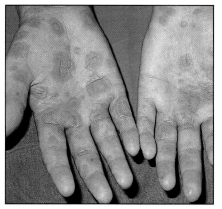

Figure 56.2 *Erythema multiforme: the typical concentric rings are particularly obvious at this site.*

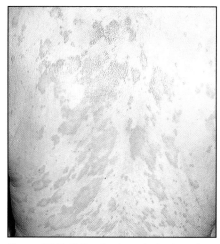

Figure 56.3 *Urticaria: irregularly shaped lesions like this are not suggestive of erythema multiforme.*

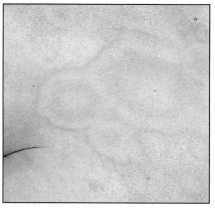

Figure 56.4 *Urticaria: there are coalescing weals with a surrounding flare, but without the concentric rings which would occur centrally in erythema multiforme.*

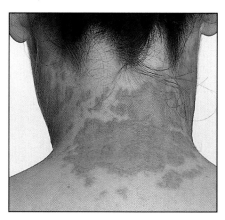

Figure 56.5 *Acute febrile neutrophilic dermatosis (Sweet's disease), a disorder which is particularly associated with infections and haematological disorders. Inflammatory and sometimes annular lesions may be confused with erythema multiforme.*

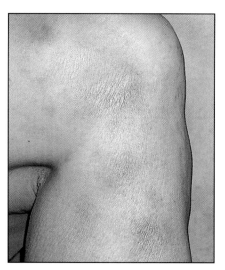

Figure 56.6 *Erythema nodosum (post-streptococcal): early lesions are sometimes confused with erythema multiforme but usually affect the legs and are typically deep and tender.*

Further reading:
p. 24, p. 42, p. 80, p. 100, p. 104, p. 114, p. 142, p. 168.

References
Champion RH, Highet AS. Investigation and management of chronic urticaria and angioedema. *Clin Exp Dermatol* 1982; **7**:291–300.
Drago F, Parodi A, Rebora A. Persistent erythema multiforme: report of two new cases and review of literature. *J Am Acad Dermatol* 1995; **33**:366–9.

Huff JC, *et al*. Erythema multiforme: a critical review of characteristics, diagnostic criteria, and causes. *J Am Acad Dermatol* 1983; **8**:763–75.
Imamura S, *et al*. Erythema multiforme. Pathomechanism of papular erythema and target lesion. *J Dermatol* 1992; **19**:524–33.

Common presenting feature: both disorders may present as an itchy eczematous eruption.

Rationale for comparison: bullous pemphigoid may have an early 'pre-pemphigoid' phase which has eczematous morphology but no blistering. An increasingly severe eczematous rash in an elderly patient may be the precursor of potentially severe generalized blistering caused by bullous pemphigoid.

Other differential diagnoses: urticaria; scabies; pemphigus (p. 116); dermatitis herpetiformis (p. 108); excoriations due to pruritus of various causes; epidermolysis bullosa acquisita; papuloerythroderma.

Conclusion and key points: in its early phase, pemphigoid may produce an intensely itchy eczematous eruption, with raised red inflammatory plaques (which are termed 'urticated' because they resemble urticaria, though they are relatively fixed in position and last for days or weeks). Bullous pemphigoid should therefore be suspected if a severe progressive eczematous eruption occurs as a new development in any elderly individual. Skin biopsy with immunofluorescence is the appropriate investigation. The diagnosis should be confirmed in this way because of the potential requirement for long-term high-dose systemic corticosteroid and immunosuppressive therapy.

Comparative features		
Disorder	**Bullous pemphigoid**	**Eczema**
Age	Mostly >70 yrs	Any
Sex	Either	
Family history	Negative	Depends on type of eczema. Mostly non-specific, but may be positive in late onset atopics.
Sites	Trunk, limbs. Facial or intraoral lesions are uncommon.	Any, not mucosal
Symptoms	Itch	
Signs common to both	Itchy, urticated, sometimes annular, plaques, excoriations, and crusting. Palmar pompholyx vesicles occur in either disorder.	
Discriminatory signs	Large unilocular blisters, often haemorrhagic, arise on either the abnormal or on clinically normal skin. More oedematous 'urticated' lesions are present than in eczemas; chronic features such as lichenification are uncommon.	Weeping/crusted lesions may occur, especially in discoid eczema, but frank blistering is rare. Lichenification may occur in more chronic lesions.
Associated features	Mouth involvement occurs in 5% of cases. There is a debatable increased frequency of internal malignancy, but blind screening is not warranted.	Eosinophilia is common in elderly patients with eczema, but also occurs in pemphigoid. May be other long-standing atopic features, e.g. asthma
Important tests	Skin biopsy with direct immunofluorescence. Baseline blood tests in anticipation of high dose systemic corticosteroid and immunosuppressive treatment.	Depends on the pattern of eczema. Relevant tests may include IgE level to support a diagnosis of atopic dermatitis (this disorder may be difficult to identify with confidence when onset is in older patients), patch tests for external contact allergens, and skin biopsy with immunofluorescence if the diagnosis is uncertain.

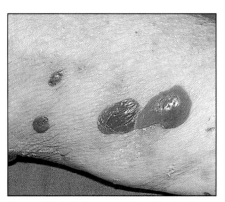

Figure 57.1 *Bullous pemphigoid, showing unilocular haemorrhagic blisters arising on non-inflamed skin.*

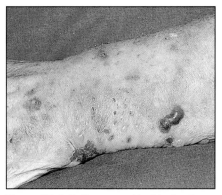

Figure 57.2 *Bullous pemphigoid, showing unilocular blisters with either clear fluid or blood-stained fluid content, arising on an eczematous background.*

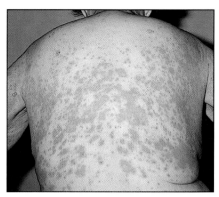

Figure 57.3 *Pre-pemphigoid, showing 'urticated' plaques which may be confused with eczema in an elderly patient.*

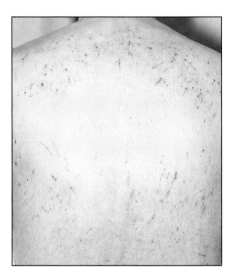

Figure 57.4 *Eczematized skin due to scratching in a patient with pruritus. Note that the central 'butterfly area' of the back is spared as the patient cannot reach this area to scratch it—sparing of this area would not be expected when the skin eruption is endogenous (compare with Fig. 57.3 and Fig. 54.5).*

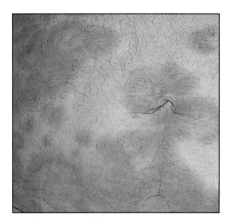

Figure 57.5 *Annular lesions are a frequent pattern in the pre-bullous stage of pemphigoid.*

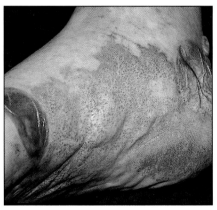

Figure 57.6 *Plantar vesicles in bullous pemphigoid. This pompholyx appearance usually occurs as a type of eczema, but is also found in 25% of patients with bullous pemphigoid (see also p. 66).*

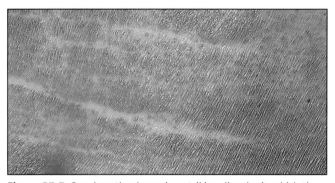

Figure 57.7 *Papuloerythroderma is a striking disorder in which there are extensive sheets of semiconfluent papules with sparing of skin creases as shown here. Clinically, it may behave as a form of eczema, especially in elderly men, and may therefore be included in the differential diagnosis of eczema or pre-pemphigoid.*

Further reading:
p. 66, p. 94, p. 108, p. 112, p. 116, p. 142, p. 144.

References
Duhra P, Ryatt KS. Haemorrhagic pompholyx in bullous pemphigoid. *Clin Exp Dermatol* 1988; **13**:342–3.
Frain Bell W. Bullous dermatitis and bullous pemphigoid. *Br J Dermatol* 1959; **71**:241–6.
Haustein UF. Bullous scabies. *Dermatology* 1995; **190**:83–4.

Korman NJ. Bullous pemphigoid. *Dermatol Clinics* 1993; **11**:483–98.
Morrison LH, Diaz LA, Anhalt GJ. Bullous pemphigoid. In: Wojnarowska F, Briggaman RA (eds). *Management of blistering disorders*. Chapman & Hall, London, 1990:63–82.
Strohal R, *et al*. Nonbullous pemphigoid: prodrome of bullous pemphigoid or a distinct pemphigoid variant? *J Am Acad Dermatol* 1993; **29**:293–9.

Common presenting feature: itchy eczematous eruption, blisters.

Rationale for comparison: these disorders are often confused, at least in part due to their similar names. They do, however, have a very different morphology and can usually be differentiated on clinical grounds. Both are potentially serious and require long-term systemic therapy.

Other differential diagnoses: urticaria; erythema multiforme; toxic epidermal necrolysis; staphylococcal scalded skin syndrome; eczema; scabies; other immunobullous disorders (e.g. dermatitis herpetiformis, epidermolysis bullosa acquisita).

Conclusion and key points: there are two main variants of pemphigus. Pemphigus foliaceous causes very superficial fragile blisters that burst easily; this variant therefore generally presents as a series of crusted lesions which may be confused with eczema and fungal infection. In pemphigus vulgaris, the blisters occur at a deeper level within the epidermis; the patient usually presents with large erosions, sometimes with intact flaccid blisters, and typically with preceding or concomitant mouth ulceration. Bleeding into the blisters is not a typical feature of pemphigus, as the damage in both variants is within the epidermis, which does not contain blood vessels. In bullous pemphigoid, the blisters occur between the epidermis and the dermis, and the epidermis is not specifically damaged; the blister roof is therefore stronger and thicker and the clinical appearance is of tense, unilocular, haemorrhagic blisters. Skin biopsy with immunofluorescence of uninvolved perilesional skin is the appropriate investigation to differentiate these disorders and is important in view of their requirement for aggressive systemic therapy.

Comparative features		
Disorder	**Bullous pemphigoid**	**Pemphigus**
Age	Mostly >70 yrs	Mostly 50–60 yrs
Sex	Either	
Family history	Negative	
Sites	Trunk and limbs. Facial or intraoral lesions are uncommon.	Any site. Pemphigus foliaceous is predominantly truncal and facial. Pemphigus vulgaris typically involves mucosae, usually several weeks or months before development of skin lesions.
Symptoms	Itch; pain when blisters burst to leave an eroded base	Itch; pain due to skin erosions. Oral erosions are painful.
Signs common to both	Itchy plaques, erosions, fragile blisters, crusting. Oral mucosal blisters and/or erosions	
Discriminatory signs	Large unilocular blisters, often haemorrhagic, which arise on either the abnormal 'urticated' skin or on clinically normal skin	Erosions and crusted lesions are typical as blisters are flaccid and fragile. Frank blistering also occurs, particularly in pemphigus vulgaris.
Associated features	Mouth involvement occurs in 5% of cases, and is usually mild.	Oral lesions are typical of pemphigus vulgaris (80–90%); ocular and vaginal mucosal involvement may also be present.
Important tests	Skin biopsy with direct immunofluorescence demonstrates IgG and C3 in a linear band at the basement membrane zone. Baseline blood tests for potential high dose systemic corticosteroid treatment	Skin biopsy with direct immunofluorescence demonstrates intercellular IgG and C3 within the epidermis. Deposits along the basement membrane zone as well as between keratinocytes occurs in paraneoplastic pemphigus. Baseline blood tests for potential high dose systemic corticosteroid treatment

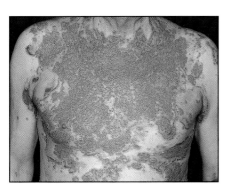

Figure 58.1
Pemphigus, showing widespread erosions and crusting without prominent intact blisters.

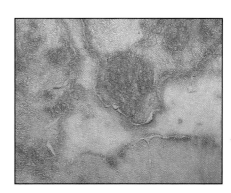

Figure 58.2
Pemphigus: closer view of erosions and crusting.

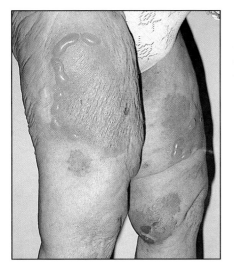

Figure 58.3
Pemphigoid: there are tense clear blisters with annular arrangement.

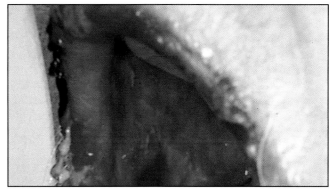

Figure 58.4 *Pemphigus vulgaris: oral lesions often precede skin blistering by a few months. Due to the fragile nature of mucosal surfaces, and trauma from eating, it is very uncommon to see intact blisters—the usual feature is widespread erosions.*

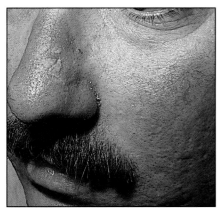

Figure 58.5 *Pemphigus foliaceous: nasal crusting reminiscent of seborrhoeic dermatitis is a fairly common (and occasionally the only) feature.*

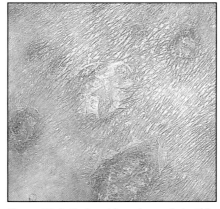

Figure 58.6 *Toxic epidermal necrolysis: this is a severe pattern of drug eruption that may be morphologically indistinguishable from pemphigus.*

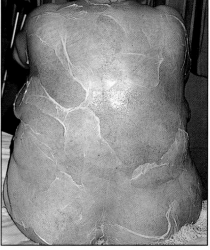

Figure 58.7 *Staphylococcal scalded skin syndrome: this generally produces much larger sheets of skin shedding.*

Further reading:
p. 66, p. 108, p. 112, p. 114, p. 142, p. 144.

References

Huilgol SC, Black MM. Management of the immunobullous disorders. II. Pemphigus. *Clin Exp Dermatol* 1995; **20**:283–93.

Muller S, Stanley JR. Pemphigus: pemphigus vulgaris and pemphigus foliaceous. In: Wojnarowska F, Briggaman RA (eds). *Management of blistering disorders*. Chapman & Hall, London, 1990:43–61.

Rosenberg FR, Sanders S, Nelson G. Pemphigus. *Arch Dermatol* 1976; **112**:962–70.

Savin JA. The events leading to death of patients with pemphigus and pemphigoid. *Br J Dermatol* 1979; **101**:521–34.

Common presenting feature: both disorders cause a confluent erythematous flexural rash.

Rationale for comparison: the two diagnoses have different therapeutic and investigative implications.

Other differential diagnoses: tinea (p. 120); erythrasma; Hailey–Hailey disease; intertrigo; *Candida* infection; contact allergy; vulval dystrophy/malignancy; lichen sclerosus et atrophicus (p. 124); lichen planus; extramammary Paget's disease; threadworm infestation.

Conclusion and key points: in many instances, the treatment of flexural eczema or psoriasis is similar. However, it is important to differentiate eczema because there may be specific causative or contributary contact allergies. Additionally, some treatments which are suitable for flexural psoriasis (e.g. mild tar preparations) are not usually appropriate for eczemas. Psoriasis tends to have a more moist shiny or 'glazed' erythema and a sharper border than flexural eczemas, but lesions at other body sites may be the best discriminator. Several of the differential diagnoses listed also have important therapeutic differences.

Genital (as opposed to flexural) rash is a common diagnostic and therapeutic problem in either sex. In women, vulval discomfort with a burning quality (known as vulvodynia) may occur in skin which appears normal or only slightly red. In men, an itchy scrotum is often incorrectly assumed to be of fungal origin (tinea is generally flexural rather than scrotal). Many cases of chronic genital itch involve some degree of lichen simplex, in which the skin is thickened by rubbing; exaggerated skin markings are the important physical sign of lichen simplex.

Comparative features		
Disorder	**Flexural eczema**	**Flexural psoriasis**
Age	Any. Most diagnostic and therapeutic problems arise in adults.	Psoriasis of flexures without lesions at other sites is a common distribution in children, but is uncommon in adults.
Sex	Either	
Family history	May be positive for atopy	May be positive
Sites	Atopic dermatitis of flexures is rarely a diagnostic problem. Isolated axillary eczema is often due to contact allergy (deodorants etc.), while eczema of anterior and posterior axillary folds with sparing of the apex of the axilla suggests a clothing dermatitis. Lichen simplex is a common form of perineal eczema which usually affects vulva or mons pubis in women, or scrotum and adjacent base of penis in men.	Usually symmetrical involvement of axillae and groin flexures, and genitalia. In adults, the sites may be more localized; gluteal fold involvement may be the only flexural psoriasis present, but other solitary localized sites may be affected, such as the glans penis in men.
Symptoms	Itch	None, itch
Signs common to both	Confluent erythema. In either disorder, the degree of scaling is less than that typically present at extraflexural sites.	
Discriminatory signs	Usually pinkish-red, often slightly ill-defined border. Lichen simplex of genital skin causes exaggerated skin markings.	Often bright 'pillar-box' red with a glazed surface, and typically a sharply demarcated border
Associated features	There may be lesions at other sites, but eczema may be localized to the involved flexure(s) only (e.g. deodorant reactions are limited to the axilla).	There are usually lesions at other sites also; pure flexural psoriasis is relatively unusual. Umbilical involvement is common when the flexures are affected.
Important tests	Patch test (especially fragrances, deodorants etc.). In genital and perineal skin, asymmetrical 'eczema' may need biopsy to exclude extramammary Paget's disease.	None usually, but biopsy may be needed if the diagnosis is uncertain, especially if the vulva or glans penis is the only site affected.

Causes of perineal or genital eczema

Primary irritant	Faecal leakage, laxatives, soaps
Lichen simplex	Especially scrotal, vulval, mons pubis
Contact allergy	Fragrances, local anaesthetics, antibiotics, antifungals, corticosteroids, other constituents of topical creams
Seborrhoeic	Usually other sites also affected

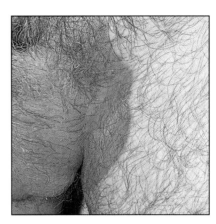

Figure 59.1
Psoriasis of the groin flexure in a man: this is a common site. Note the beefy-red colour and sharply demarcated border.

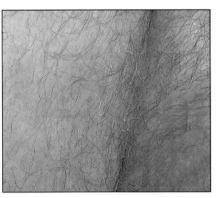

Figure 59.2 *Intertriginous rash in the groin of a man: there is somewhat eczematous morphology, which was aggravated by sweating. Skin scrapings identified corynebacteria.*

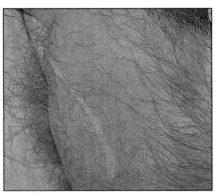

Figure 59.3 *Lichen simplex of the scrotum, showing erythema and exaggerated skin markings.*

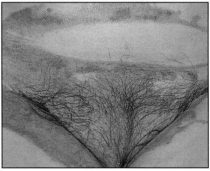

Figure 59.4 *Flexural skin staining by codanthromer (a laxative) excreted in stools: the rather brown colour is typical. The irregular angulated shapes and sparing of the deeper part of the flexures identify this eruption as having an exogenous cause.*

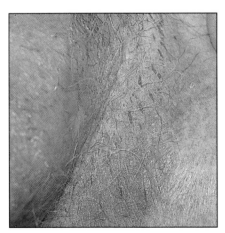

Figure 59.5
Hailey–Hailey disease, an autosomal dominant disorder of the flexures. It produces rather eczematous and fairly discrete plaques with apparent small tears in the surface, which appear as red linear marks among the whiter macerated keratin.

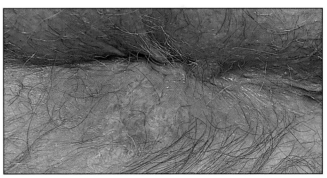

Figure 59.6 *Extramammary Paget's disease may resemble eczema, but is due to an underlying carcinoma which may arise from skin appendages or from the rectal mucosa. The perianal area is a typical site; the relative lack of itch, progressive skin abnormality, and often asymmetry around the anus, are useful features which help to distinguish it from the much more common irritant pruritus ani.*

Further reading:
p. 2, p. 26, p. 28, pp. 58–64, p. 82, p. 102, p. 110, p. 120, p. 126, p. 174, p. 176.

References
Burge SM. Hailey–Hailey disease. Clinical features, response to treatment and prognosis. *Br J Dermatol* 1992; **126**:275–82.
McKay M. Vulvar manifestation of skin disorders (non-neoplastic epithelial disorders). In: Black MM, McKay M, Braude P (eds). *Color atlas and text of obstetric and gynecologic dermatology.* Mosby–Wolfe, London, 1995:91–100.
Ridley CM, Oriel JD, Robinson AJ. *A colour atlas of diseases of the vulva.* London, Chapman & Hall.1992.

Common presenting feature: sharply demarcated erythematous flexural rash.

Rationale for comparison: different treatment is required for these clinically distinguishable conditions.

Other differential diagnoses: lichen simplex and other eczema (see p. 118); intertrigo; erythrasma; *Candida* infection; Hailey–Hailey disease (Fig. 59.5); extramammary Paget's disease (Fig. 59.6); axillary eruptions (e.g. freckling in neurofibromatosis [Crowe's sign, Fig. 82.8]; pseudoxanthoma elasticum, Fox–Fordyce disease).

Conclusion and key points: this differential diagnostic problem arises most commonly in the perineal area and groin flexures. Concurrent involvement of the axillae is common in psoriasis, erythrasma and Hailey–Hailey disease but is extremely uncommon in tinea infections. Tinea usually has marginal accentuation and fine scale compared with the more confluent erythema and moist surface of flexural psoriasis. Where doubt exists, scrapings should be taken for mycological examination from any affected sites. The feet should be specifically examined as tinea pedis or toenail fungal infection is almost invariably present in individuals with groin or perineal tinea infection.

Comparative features		
Disorder	**Flexural psoriasis**	**Tinea**
Age	Mainly child or young adult onset	Adult, especially younger age group
Sex	Either	Strong male predominance; associated with higher prevalence of tinea pedis in men
Family history	May be positive	Non-specific
Sites	Usually affects both axillae and groin flexures	Perineal and groin flexures; rare in axillae
Symptoms	None, itch	
Signs common to both	Sharply demarcated symmetrical erythema with some scaling	
Discriminatory signs	The degree of erythema is even throughout the lesion; there is often quite a deep red colour, and a 'glazed' or moist surface. There may be more typical psoriatic scale if the plaque extends beyond the apposed skin of the flexural area. Psoriasis often affects the gluteal fold in either sex, and the penis and scrotum in men. When the groin area is affected there is typically concurrent axillary involvement also.	Gradually expanding, finely scaling patch with marginal accentuation of erythema and scaling (Figs 48.2, 48.3). Fungal infection affects flexures rather than genitalia. Usually fairly symmetrical but the border of larger areas tends to become irregular as the patch enlarges
Associated features	May affect other body sites also; typically elbows, knees, scalp, nails	Typically there is also toeweb, plantar, or toenail involvement.
Important tests	None	Examine the feet. Skin scrapings for mycology (Figs 55.6, 55.7).

Further reading:
p. 2, pp. 58–64, p. 82, p. 102, p. 110, p. 118, p. 126, p. 174, p. 176.

References
Odom R. Pathophysiology of dermatophyte infections. *J Am Acad Dermatol* 1993; **28**:52–7.

Rezabek GH, Friedman AD. Superficial fungal infections of the skin. Diagnosis and current treatment recommendations. *Drugs* 1992; **43**:674–82.

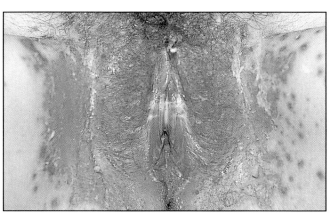

Figure 60.1 *Acute flexural psoriasis: similar erythema and 'satellite' lesions are seen in genital and perineal candidal infections.*

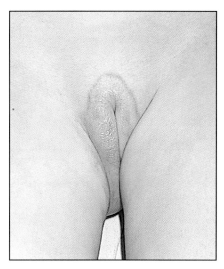

Figure 60.2
Psoriasis of the vulva in a child: this does have a prominent margin but is very symmetrical. In addition, tinea cruris would be highly unusual in a girl of this age.

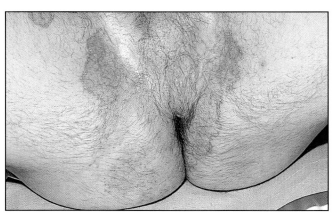

Figure 60.3 *Tinea cruris: note the spreading irregularly shaped border.*

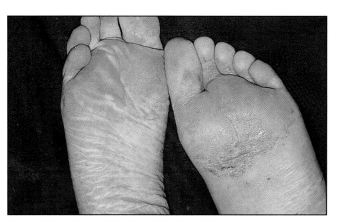

Figure 60.4 *Fungal infection of the feet: this is almost always identifiable in patients with tinea in the groin or perineum.*

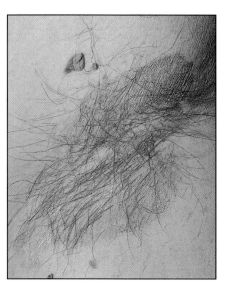

Figure 60.5
Erythrasma: this corynebacterial infection resembles tinea but has a browner colour and lacks any marginal accentuation.

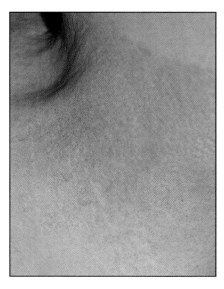

Figure 60.6
Pseudoxanthoma elasticum: this is an inherited defect of elastic fibres which produces a 'plucked chicken' appearance, mainly affecting the axillae and neck (illustrated here).

Common presenting feature: nappy rash in infancy.

Rationale for comparison: these two disorders may coexist, but their treatments and prognoses are different.

Other differential diagnoses: more general forms of dermatitis affecting the nappy area (atopic, seborrhoeic); psoriasis; other infections (e.g. impetigo); rarer eruptions (e.g. histiocytosis X, acrodermatitic enteropathica due to zinc deficiency).

Conclusion and key points: *Candida albicans* commonly infects or colonizes any nappy rash in infants. It is also a primary cause of skin eruption at this site, and is characterized by the presence of a beefy-red rash, pustules, and scattered 'satellite' lesions outside the main confluent part of the eruption. Examination of the mouth should be carried out in babies with a possible candidal nappy rash as this may demonstrate oral candidosis. Treatment of the mouth and gastrointestinal tract is helpful as the nappy rash may otherwise recur after topical treatment.

Comparative features

Disorder	Nappy dermatitis	Candidosis
Age	Infant	
Sex	Either	
Family history	Non-specific	
Sites	Nappy area. An irritant dermatitis characteristically spares the creases and is localized to the nappy area, while seborrhoeic dermatitis involves all the flexures and extends to other areas of the body (especially scalp and axillae).	Nappy area. Typically includes the creases
Symptoms	None, itch, pain (irritant type with soiled nappies)	Discomfort
Signs common to both	Erythematous rash in nappy area; may be moist/oozing surface	
Discriminatory signs	Irritant: flexural sparing Seborrhoeic: more orange colour; scattered lesions on trunk with yellowish-brown scale; presence of cradle cap of scalp; relative lack of symptoms apparent by lack of distress	Beefy-red colour; flexural involvement; presence of pustules and satellite lesions
Associated features	Irritant type: may be atopic dermatitis elsewhere Seborrhoeic: rash elsewhere, especially cradle cap	Oral lesions of *Candida* (p. 18)
Important tests	None; bacteriology swabs if uncertainty	Bacteriology swabs, mouth and nappy area

Further reading:
p. 18, p. 26, p. 130.

References
Bodey GP. *Candidiasis. Pathogenesis, diagnosis and treatment*, 2nd edn. Raven Press, New York, 1993.
Judge MR, McDonald A, Black MM. Pustular psoriasis in childhood. *Clin Exp Dermatol* 1993; **18**:97–9.
Loughi F, *et al*. Diaper dermatitis: a study of contributing factors. *Contact Dermatitis* 1992; **26**:248–52.
Robinson AJ, Ridgwat GL. Sexually transmitted diseases in children. *Genitourin Med* 1994; **70**:208–14.

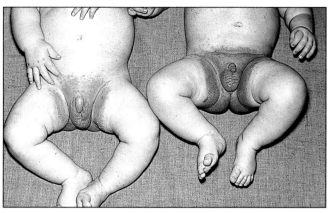

Figure 61.1 *Severe irritant dermatitis of the nappy area in siblings, demonstrating relatively sharp demarcation and flexural sparing (photograph kindly provided by Dr W. D. Paterson).*

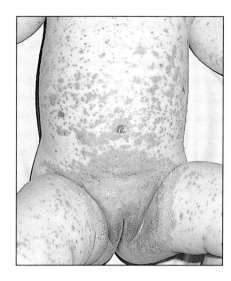

Figure 61.2
Infantile seborrhoeic dermatitis with predominant involvement of the nappy area (see also Fig. 13.1).

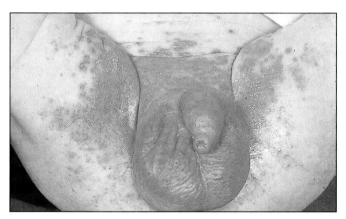

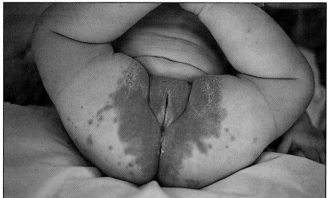

Figures 61.3 and 61.4 *Examples of* Candida albicans *infection of the nappy area, demonstrating confluent erythema and satellite lesions beyond the main area of the eruption.*

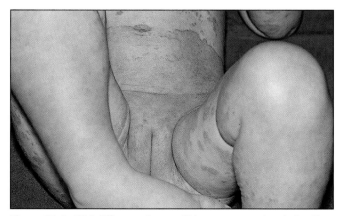

Figure 61.5 *Mild diffuse erythema of the nappy area in a baby: the relatively pale colour and accentuated margin excluded candidosis, but a clear distinction between seborrhoeic dermatitis and infantile psoriasis could not be determined.*

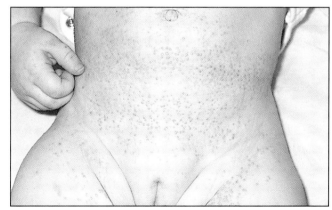

Figure 61.6 *Extensive papular eruption centred around the nappy area in an infant. This caused concern about possible histiocytosis X, but this proved to be a transient eruption associated with symptoms of a viral respiratory infection.*

Genital lichen sclerosus in women v. dermatitis

Common presenting feature: itchy vulval or perianal rash in women.

Rationale for comparison: therapeutic and prognostic differences.

Other differential diagnoses: other vulval dystrophies and neoplasia; lichen planus; Hailey–Hailey disease; psoriasis (pp. 118–120); lichen simplex; intertrigo; tinea; vitiligo; *Candida* infection; threadworm infestation (perianal itch mainly); sexual abuse in children.

Conclusion and key points: lichen sclerosus is relatively common and may be an incidental asymptomatic finding (in which case it is unlikely to be confused with dermatitis). It commonly causes diagnostic problems when patients present with itch. Characteristic features are smooth white vulval or perivulval and perianal skin, in a pattern which is described as a 'figure 8 distribution'. There may be some degree of purpura because the inflammatory process damages collagen and reduces the support of the dermal blood vessels. Sclerosis causes abnormal vulval architecture, such as fusion of labia minora, urethral stenosis, and vaginal stenosis (and hence dyspareunia). Potent topical corticosteroid therapy is indicated, and there is a long-term risk of squamous cell carcinoma, hence the importance of recognizing this condition.

The distinction between lichen sclerosis and other inflammatory dermatoses in men is rarely a problem. Lichen sclerosis affects the glans penis and the prepuce and causes white areas known as balanitis xerotica obliterans. Male patients present because of the colour change or phimosis, rather than due to itch.

Comparative features		
Disorder	**Genital lichen sclerosus in women**	**Vulval dermatitis**
Age	Any. Most patients present around the menopause, but a significant minority are children.	Adult
Sex	Either. Since lichen sclerosus is unlikely to be confused with dermatitis in men, however, only vulval lichen sclerosus is described here.	
Family history	May be positive (including identical and non-identical twins)	Non-specific
Sites	Figure-of-8 pattern encircling the vulval and perianal skin, connected at the perineum	Vulval, perineal, perianal
Symptoms	None, itch, dyspareunia, or difficulty with micturition	Always symptomatic of itch or discomfort
Signs common to both	Swelling, lichenification, erosions. However, early lichen sclerosus, although usually pale in colour, is not atrophic or scarring and may be confused with dermatitis. Established lichen sclerosus is generally clinically characteristic and unlikely to be confused with dermatitis, although both disorders may present as vulval itch.	
Discriminatory signs	Alteration of vulval architecture due to scarring, especially atrophy of labia minora and fusion of labia minora or majora causing stenosis of the introitus. There is a pale ivory-white colour, purpuric areas, and sometimes small haemorrhagic blisters.	Lichenification, erythema and scaling rather than pallor. The edge of the affected area is often poorly demarcated.
Associated features	There may be extragenital lichen sclerosus et atrophicus (p. 92)	There may be dermatitis elsewhere.
Important tests	Biopsy may be required to support the diagnosis, or to exclude vulval intraepithelial neoplasia.	Patch testing
Complications	Urethral or vulval stenosis, squamous cell carcinoma in 5% of known cases. Childhood lichen sclerosus usually resolves spontaneously.	

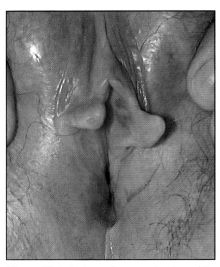

Figure 62.1 *Lichen sclerosus, showing white colour, erosions, and loss of labia minora, intriotal stenosis.*

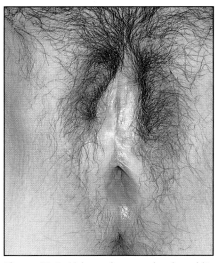

Figure 62.2 *Lichen sclerosus, showing white colour, labial fusion, and introital stenosis.*

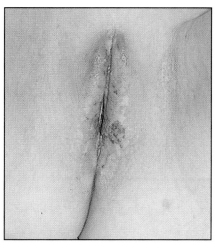

Figure 62.3 *Lichen sclerosus in a child: the patient was referred to the paediatric department because the lesion had raised concern of sexual abuse. The white colour and purpuric component are typical of lichen sclerosus.*

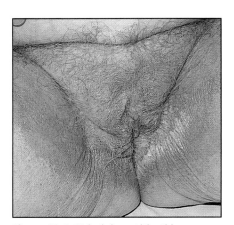

Figure 62.4 *Vulval dermatitis: this was a contact reaction to a fragrance in cream the patient was applying.*

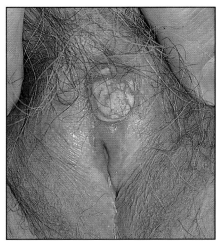

Figure 62.5 *Squamous cell carcinoma of vulva: this is a potential complication of lichen sclerosus.*

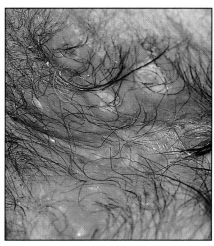

Figure 62.6 *Perianal ulceration in a patient having chemotherapy: this healed with simple antiseptic and barrier preparations and was presumably due to infection of macerated skin. Other causes of multiple perineal ulcers include herpes simplex, cytomegalovirus, candidosis, inflammatory bowel disease, fixed drug eruption, immunobullous disorders and lichen planus or lichen sclerosus.*

Further reading:
p. 92, p. 110, p. 118, p. 120.

References
Chanco Turner ML. Management of lichen sclerosus. In: Dahl MV (ed). *Curr Opin Dermatol* 1996; **3**:3–9.

Krafchik BR. Advances in vulvar disease: lichen sclerosus et atrophicus. *Adv Dermatol* 1992; **7**:163–77.

McKay M. Vulvar manifestation of skin disorders (non-neoplastic epithelial disorders). In: Black MM, McKay M, Braude P (eds). *Color atlas and text of obstetric and gynecologic dermatology*. Mosby–Wolfe, London, 1995:91–100.

Neill SM. Vulvar lichen sclerosus. In: Black MM, McKay M, Braude P. *Color atlas and text of obsteric and gynecologic dermatology*. Mosby–Wolfe, London 1995:119–24.

Ridley CM. Genital lichen sclerosus (lichen sclerosus et atrophicus) in childhood and adolescence. *J Roy Soc Med* 1993; **86**:69–75.

Common presenting feature: erythematous rash affecting the glans penis.

Rationale for comparison: different causes and therapeutic options.

Other differential diagnoses: candidosis or other infection; Reiter's syndrome; lichen planus; erythroplasia of Queyrat (penile Bowen's disease); extramammary Paget's disease; squamous cell carcinoma.

Conclusion and key points: Zoon's balanitis produces a well-defined reddish-brown plaque on the glans penis and foreskin. This characteristically has a lobulated shape and glazed moist surface and is usually clinically identifiable. However, it may be confused with psoriasis, and more importantly with Bowen's disease of the penis (erythroplasia of Queyrat). Zoon's balanitis often responds to topical antibiotics, or to topical corticosteroids, but circumcision may be required in some cases.

Comparative features		
Disorder	**Penile psoriasis**	**Zoon's balanitis**
Age	Any; confusion arises in adults rather than in children.	Adult
Sex	Male	
Family history	May be positive	Non-specific
Sites	Any part of penis. The main diagnostic concerns relate to isolated psoriasis of the glans penis.	Glans penis and foreskin in uncircumcised men
Symptoms	May be itchy in adults	Often none; may be soreness due to moist surface adhering to clothing
Signs common to both	Erythematous localized plaque	
Discriminatory signs	Bright red colour; often variable severity over a period of time; may be rather annular morphology	Dusky red-purple colour; confluent lesion with lobulated margin
Associated features	May be psoriasis elsewhere	None
Important tests	Biopsy if diagnostic doubt	Biopsy may be required to exclude neoplasia; bacteriology swabs
Treatment	Topical corticosteroids; may include an imidazole or antiseptic to prevent candidal overgrowth	Topical anti-staphylococcal antibiotics, imidazoles, corticosteroids; treatments to dry moist surface (e.g. potassium permanganate soaks), circumcision

Further reading:
p. 118, p. 120.

References
Camisa C. *Psoriasis*. Blackwell Scientific Publications, Boston, 1994:53–83.

Souteyrand P, Wong E, MacDonald DM. Zoon's balanitis (balanitis circumscripta plasmacellularis). *Br J Dermatol* 1981; **105**:195–9.

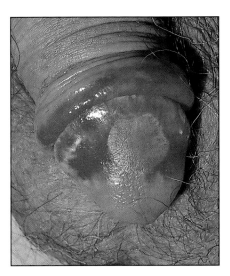

Figure 63.1 *Zoon's balanitis, showing typical moist bright-red surface, involving the glans penis and prepuce.*

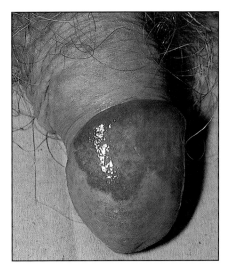

Figure 63.2 *Zoon's balanitis, showing typical moist bright-red surface and lobulated shape.*

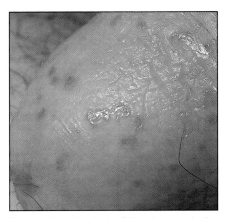

Figure 63.3 *Psoriasis of the glans penis, in this case with multiple small lesions.*

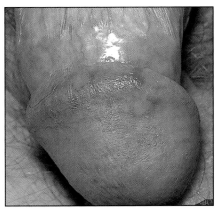

Figure 63.4 *Circinate balanitis, in a man with ankylosing spondylitis.*

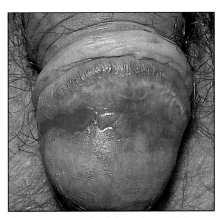

Figure 63.5 *Erosive lichen planus of the glans penis closely resembling Zoon's balanitis.*

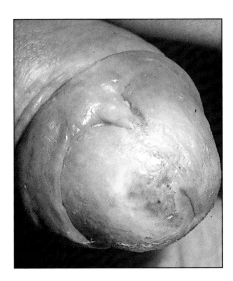

Figure 63.6 *Lichen sclerosus (balanitis xerotica obliterans): demonstrating white colour, purpura, and scarring of foreskin.*

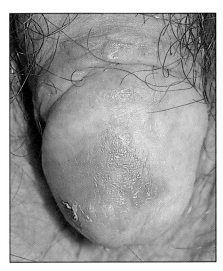

Figure 63.7 *Bowen's disease of the penis: this may be confused with psoriasis but slowly increases in size, whereas psoriasis is variable in its clinical course.*

Common presenting feature: penile or vulval lesions, usually multiple.

Rationale for comparison: bowenoid papulosis is particularly associated with a viral wart type (human papillomavirus [HPV] 16) which carries a much higher risk of malignancy than do the more common genital wart HPV types 6 and 11.

Other differential diagnoses: sebaceous gland hyperplasia of penis/vulva; penile pearly papules; cysts of vulva/scrotum; molluscum contagiosum; scabies nodules (Fig. 53.6); Bowen's disease/erythroplasia of Queyrat (Fig. 63.7); squamous cell carcinoma; fibroepithelial polyps; angiokeratomas of scrotum/vulva.

Conclusion and key points: bowenoid papulosis and genital viral warts have a similar morphology, but can usually be differentiated by the presence of brown or grey pigmentation in bowenoid papulosis. Both disorders may occur in either sex. Although bowenoid papulosis lesions have histological features of Bowen's disease (and are therefore classified as a form of vulval intraepithelial neoplasia, VIN) they may sometimes be non-progressive, or even spontaneously regress. However, they are strongly associated with HPV 16 infection and therefore identify a group of patients with a higher risk of genital neoplasia compared with patients who have had common genital warts of HPV type 6 or 11. In those who do develop a neoplasm, this may be vulval or cervical, and not specifically related to the sites of bowenoid papulosis lesions. Regular examination and cervical smear (in women) is therefore appropriate for patients who have, or have had, bowenoid papulosis. Normal structures, such as sebaceous glands, may sometimes be mistaken for warts and inappropriately treated.

Comparative features		
Disorder	**Viral wart**	**Bowenoid papulosis**
Age	Young adult	
Sex	Either, usually more obvious in male	
Family history	Non-specific but partner usually clinically affected	
Sites	Male: Penis, perianal region Female: Vulva, vagina/cervix, perianal region	
Symptoms	Usually none	
Signs common to both	Warty nodules, usually multiple	
Discriminatory signs	Pale colour, verrucous surface	Brown or grey colour, often flatter morphology
Associated features	Uncertain risk of neoplasia, but commoner types due to HPV 6 or 11 certainly have lower risk than HPV 16 or 18	Risk of vulval or cervical neoplasia as they are usually related to HPV 16 infection
Important tests	Consider other sexually transmitted infections. In children, consider sexual abuse (see p. 130).	Follow-up examinations and cervical smear test in women

Further reading:
p. 72, p. 130, p. 178.

References
Massmanian A, *et al.* Fordyce spots on the glans penis. *Br J Dermatol* 1995; **133**:498–500.
Micali G, *et al.* Squamous cell carcinoma of the penis. *J Am Acad Dermatol* 1996; **35**:432–51.*

Rudlinger R. Bowenoid papulosis of male and female genital tracts: risk of cervical neoplasia. *J Am Acad Dermatol* 1987; **16**:625–7.
Schwartz RA, Janniger CK. Bowenoid papulosis. *J Am Acad Dermatol* 1991; **24**:261–4.

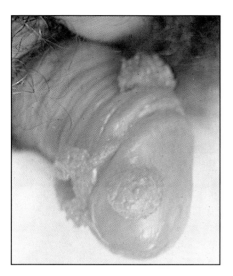

Figure 64.1 *Viral warts on the penis (photograph kindly provided by Dr R. Pattman).*

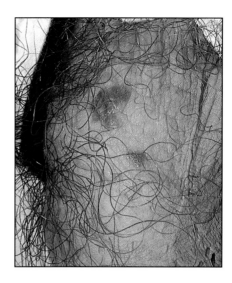

Figure 64.2 *Bowenoid papulosis on the penis, showing typical brown colour.*

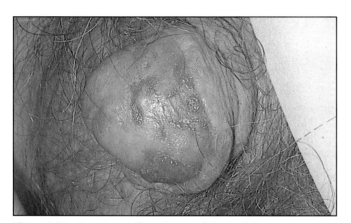

Figure 64.3 *Squamous cell carcinoma of the penis in an uncircumcised man with chronic balanitis.*

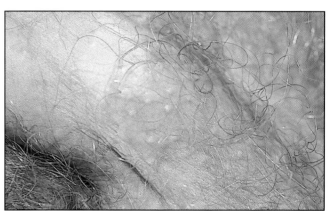

Figure 64.4 *Sebaceous hyperplasia: prominent penile sebaceous glands are sometimes mistaken for warts.*

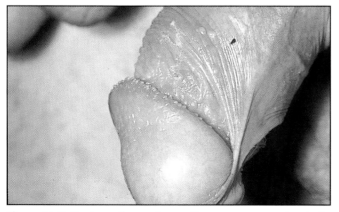

Figure 64.5 *Pearly penile papules, another common normal variant which may be mistaken for warts.*

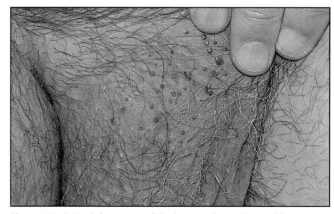

Figure 64.6 *Angiokeratoma of Fordyce on the scrotum: this may alarm patients but it is a benign condition unrelated to warts.*

Common presenting feature: perianal papules in a young child.

Rationale for comparison: different treatments. Perianal warts may occasionally occur as a result of child sexual abuse, but this is not a likely explanation for molluscum contagiosum. Correct diagnosis may therefore avoid unnecessary suspicion and investigation.

Other differential diagnoses: chickenpox (the more widespread nature of this eruption is usually apparent after a few days, but initial crops of papules may affect buttocks); epidermal naevi; condylomata lata (very rare); streptococcal infection; herpes simplex (more acute, but may cause chronic lesions in immunosuppressed patients).

Conclusion and key points: common viral warts at this site form mass lesions with a verrucous surface, whereas molluscum contagiosum lesions are individually distinct, smooth-surfaced, and umbilicated in morphology. Molluscum contagiosum lesions usually affect a broader area of the buttocks and upper thighs, and also often occur at other sites such as the axillae. Perianal and genital warts may be innocently acquired from a relative with hand warts (or during birth from a mother with genital warts), but child abuse should be considered. By contrast, molluscum contagiosum is relatively common and is usually acquired from siblings or school playmates.

Comparative features		
Disorder	**Perianal warts**	**Molluscum contagiosum**
Age	Young child	
Sex	Either	
Family history	In babies, infection may be acquired from genital warts in the mother. In infants, hand warts in a parent or carer may be a source of infection.	Other siblings may be affected.
Sites	Perianal	A more scattered distribution on buttocks, upper thighs and genital area
Symptoms	Pain due to fissures (may present as constipation)	Usually none. However, in the period of immune destruction of the lesions which occurs for a few weeks before spontaneous resolution, there may be itch, surrounding eczema, swelling, inflammation and tenderness.
Signs common to both	Papular lesions in the perianal region	
Discriminatory signs	Verrucous surface, tendency to form large masses, relatively localized	Discrete, umbilicated, rather scattered, lesions. Other sites may be affected. Lesions may become inflamed or eczematous prior to resolution.
Associated features	Look for signs of physical or sexual abuse. This is a relatively uncommon cause of perineal warts, but is more likely in older children. Hand warts in the child or parent may be a source of infection. In young babies, there may have been transmission from maternal genital tract warts during delivery; vaginal or cervical warts may not be apparent to the mother.	Often lesions at other sites, especially axillae
Important tests	Serology for sexually transmitted diseases if abuse is suspected	None

Further reading:
p. 128.

References

American Academy of Dermatology Task Force on Pediatric Dermatology. Genital warts and sexual abuse in children. *J Am Acad Dermatol* 1984; **11**:529–30.

Bunney MH, Benton EC, Cubie H. *Viral warts. Biology and treatment.* Oxford University Press, Oxford, 1992.
Raimer SS, Raimer BG. Family violence, child abuse and anogenital warts. *Arch Dermatol* 1992; **128**:842–4.

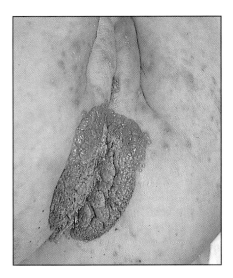

Figure 65.1 *Viral warts forming a large verrucous mass of lesions in the perianal skin.*

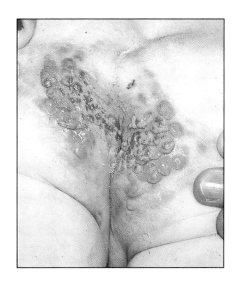

Figure 65.2 *Viral warts of the perianal skin with a rather more moist and lobulated appearance than in Fig. 65.1.*

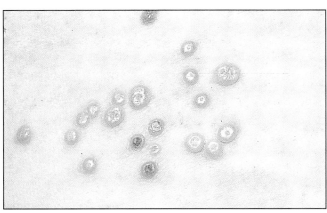

Figure 65.3 *Molluscum contagiosum, showing typical discrete smooth umbilicated grouped lesions.*

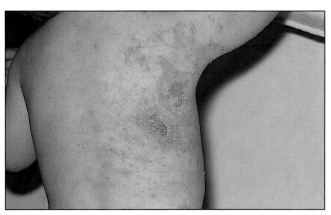

Figure 65.4 *Molluscum contagiosum in the axilla, with marked eczematization: the occurrence of itch or inflamed lesions is a common reason for presentation, but actually represents the development of immunity and impending spontaneous resolution.*

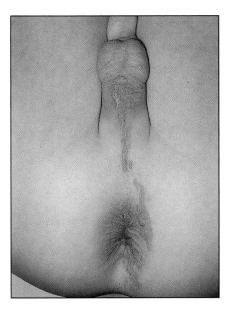

Figure 65.5 *Epidermal naevus: the perineal area is a relatively common site for this type of birthmark, which may be confused with a wart infection.*

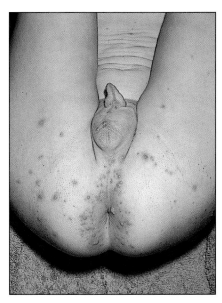

Figure 65.6 *Early chickenpox: the lesions often affect the buttock and perineal region, but are more acute in onset than perianal warts or molluscum contagiosum. The lesions are usually itchy, but may cause few symptoms in young children.*

Common presenting feature: dry, variably itchy skin lesions in children.

Rationale for comparison: commonly confused conditions which may coexist but which have therapeutic and prognostic differences.

Other differential diagnoses: bacterial folliculitis; pityrosporum folliculitis; ichthyoses; localized pityriasis rubra pilaris; digitate keratoses; lichen spinulosa.

Conclusion and key points: keratosis pilaris is a very common condition which has a typical site distribution on the outer aspect of the upper arms and thighs, and is characteristically more easily felt than seen. Mild involvement of the cheeks is common, and rarely there may be more diffuse facial involvement which can be associated with partial loss of eyebrows. It is one of the minor diagnostic criteria for atopic dermatitis, but also commonly occurs in isolation. It may be apparent in early childhood, but presentation in teenage girls is also common due to cosmetic concerns. Keratosis pilaris is frequently misdiagnosed as dermatitis and erroneously treated with corticosteroids. Although corticosteroids may occasionally be required for itch, emollients are the mainstay of treatment for this follicular variant of ichthyosis.

Comparative features		
Disorder	**Keratosis pilaris**	**Atopic dermatitis**
Age	Common in the 5–15 year age-group; may then resolve	Most cases present in the first 3 years of life
Sex	Either, most apparent in girls	Either
Family history	Often positive	Often positive for dermatitis or other atopic disorders
Sites	Mainly the outer aspect of the upper arms and thighs, but can be more extensive. Mild facial involvement is not uncommon, but a more severe form which may also affect eyebrows and cause hair loss (keratosis pilaris atrophicans facei) occurs less frequently.	In the 5–15 age-group in which confusion between these disorders is most likely, the main sites of atopic dermatitis are the antecubital and popliteal fossae.
Symptoms	None, mild itch	Itch, may be severe
Signs common to both	Dry skin, may be some erythema	
Discriminatory signs	Follicular distribution of small spiky keratoses, which are typically more easily felt than seen. There may be some perifollicular erythema, and occasionally pustules. The typical sites of involvement are usually diagnostic.	More diffuse patchy involvement with fine loose scaling. There is often a background of generally dry skin (atopic xerosis). Lichenification (Fig. 75.2) and excoriation are frequent and there may be weeping or crusting in acute phases.
Associated features	None	Other atopic skin signs, e.g. Dennie–Morgan infraorbital fold, pityriasis alba; other atopic diseases, e.g. asthma, hayfever
Important tests	None	None routinely required for diagnosis

Further reading:
p. 26, pp. 106–110, p. 136, p. 174.

References
Baden HP, Byers HR. Clinical findings, cutaneous pathology and response to therapy in 21 patients with keratosis pilaris atrophicus. *Arch Dermatol* 1994; **130**:469–75.
Hanifin JM, Rajka G. Diagnostic features of atopic dermatitis. *Acta Dermatovenereol Stockh* 1980(Suppl); **92**:44–7.
Poskitt L, Wilkinson JD. Natural history of keratosis pilaris. *Br J Dermatol* 1994; **130**:711–3.
Rothe MJ, Grant–Kels JM. Atopic dermatitis: an update. *J Am Acad Dermatol* 1996; **35**:1–13.

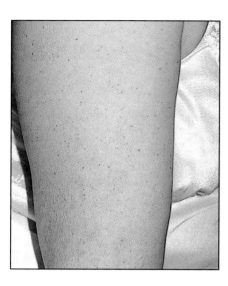

Figure 66.1
Keratosis pilaris at a typical site on the outer aspect of the upper arm.

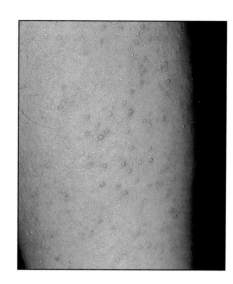

Figure 66.2
Keratosis pilaris: closer inspection reveals papular lesions and tiny follicular spikes of keratin.

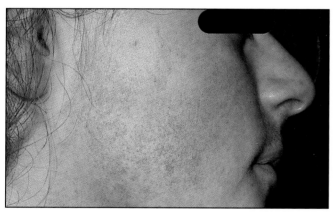

Figure 66.3 *Keratosis pilaris: diffuse facial involvement is relatively uncommon, although mild facial lesions frequently occur.*

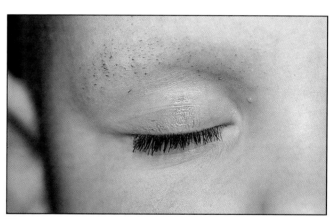

Figure 66.4 *Keratosis pilaris: eyebrow involvement with hair loss is an uncommon variant.*

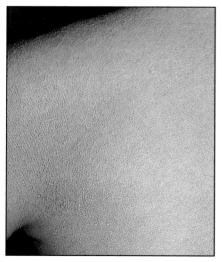

Figure 66.5 *Diffuse fine xerosis: of a type frequently associated with atopy.*

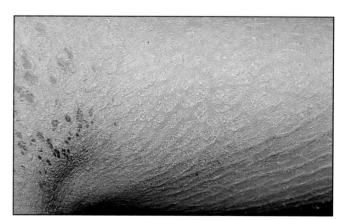

Figure 66.6 *Lamellar ichthyosis: there is a much better defined 'dirty' appearance of scaling.*

67 Psoriasis v. Bowen's disease

Common presenting feature: well-demarcated asymptomatic erythematous scaly plaque(s).

Rationale for comparison: potential diagnostic confusion may arise with only individuals having a few lesions of psoriasis. However, these conditions have totally different treatments and implications.

Other differential diagnoses: discoid eczema; lichen planus; flat seborrhoeic keratoses; actinic keratoses; squamous cell carcinoma; porokeratosis (p. 154, Fig. 77.2); dysplasia due to erythema ab igne (Fig. 77.6); basal cell carcinoma on limbs.

Conclusion and key points: if there are solitary or just a few plaques on the lower legs in elderly patients, it can be very difficult confidently to differentiate psoriasis from Bowen's disease without histological confirmation. Useful clues to suggest Bowen's disease rather than psoriasis are limitation of lesions to the lower leg, the presence of crusting rather than the silvery scale of psoriasis, and the more geographical outline of the lesions.

Comparative features		
Disorder	**Psoriasis**	**Bowen's disease**
Age	Any. Confusion with other disorders is most likely in the older age-group, as clinically atypical psoriasis is more common.	Mostly >60 yr
Sex	Either	Female predominance
Family history	May be positive	Non-specific
Sites	Any, especially extensor aspect of the limbs (on the lower legs, psoriasis usually affects the knees)	In the UK, over 80% of lesions occur on the lower leg of women; otherwise, Bowen's disease usually affects other habitually sun-exposed sites.
Symptoms	None, variable itch	Usually none, minor irritation
Signs common to both	Solitary or few well demarcated erythematous scaly plaque(s)	
Discriminatory signs	Silvery scale, which is accentuated when the surface is gently scratched (grattage, Fig. 67.2). Lesions are usually multiple and affect sites other than the leg only. Psoriasis may exhibit the Koebner reaction (localization of lesions to sites of minor injury, see Fig. 40.2).	There is crusting rather than scale, and a tendency for this to be variable at different sites within the lesion. The margin is irregular with a geographical outline. Multiple lesions occur in 25% of patients, but more than 3 or 4 lesions at any one time is unusual.
Associated features	Psoriasis at other sites, e.g. elbows, scalp, flexures, nails	If multiple lesions are present, look for signs of arsenic ingestion in the past (particularly palmar or plantar keratoses and pits).
Important tests	Usually none	Histology; may need to exclude squamous cell carcinoma
Treatment	Topical agents in most cases	Physical removal by curettage, excision, cryotherapy, sometimes radiotherapy. Topical 5-fluorouracil is helpful for multiple lesions (and has been used for psoriasis on an experimental basis).

Further reading:
p. 78, pp. 82–86, p. 102, p. 150, p. 154, p. 156.

References

Abel EA, *et al.* Drugs in exacerbations of psoriasis. *J Am Acad Dermatol* 1986; **15**:1007–22.

Chuang TY, Reisner GT. Bowen's disease and internal malignancy. *J Am Acad Dermatol* 1988; **19**:47–51.

Cox NH. Body site distribution of Bowen's disease. *Br J Dermatol* 1994; **130**:714–6.

Kossard S, Rosen R. Cutaneous Bowen's disease. An analysis of 1001 cases. *J Am Acad Dermatol* 1992; **27**:406–10.

Lee MM, Wick MM. Bowen's disease. *Clin Dermatol* 1993;**11**:43–6.

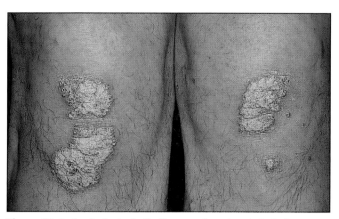

Figure 67.1 *Psoriasis: typically there are hyperkeratotic lesions on the knees. Note the closely adjacent pair of lesions on the right knee—this grouping of lesions is not a feature of Bowen's disease.*

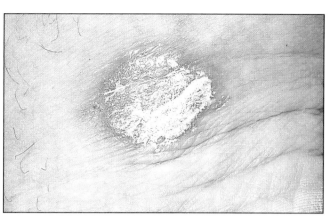

Figure 67.2 *Psoriasis: grattage (gently scratching the surface) enhances the silvery colour of the scale.*

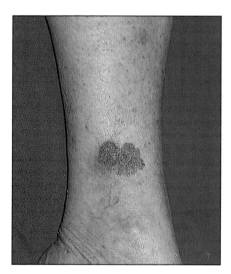

Figure 67.3 *Bowen's disease: a typical site on the lower leg.*

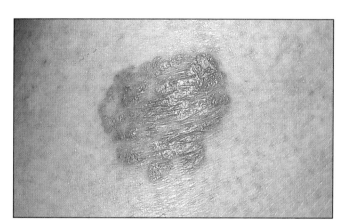

Figure 67.4 *Bowen's disease: the irregular geographical margin is typical of Bowen's disease in this relatively non-crusted lesion.*

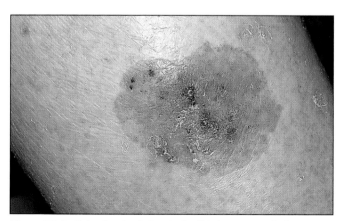

Figure 67.5 *Flat seborrhoeic keratosis: this has a very similar appearance to Bowen's disease, but the border is absolutely sharp and more lobulated and the lesion feels different upon palpation.*

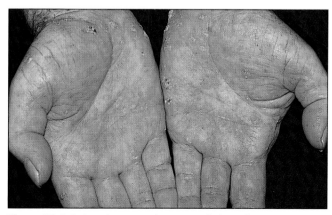

Figure 67.6 *Palmar keratoses due to arsenic ingestion as a childhood tonic: this is a frequent finding in patients with multiple lesions of Bowen's disease.*

Common presenting feature: eczematous rash of lower legs.

Rationale for comparison: the symptomatic treatment of these two conditions is similar. However, recognition of their different aetiologies offers the potential for treating the causative factors and hence preventing exacerbations.

Other differential diagnoses: ichthyoses (inherited or acquired); discoid eczema; contact allergy; vitamin C deficiency (causes purpura and residual pigmentation).

Conclusion and key points: both of these conditions are common in hospitalized elderly patients, frequently because of increased washing combined with a hot, dry environment. The 'crazy paving' morphology of asteatotic eczema is characteristic, whereas venous eczema is more diffuse and is accompanied by other signs of venous disease (dilated vessels, pigmentation, atrophie blanche). Treatment of either condition includes topical corticosteroids (initially), reducing the frequency of washing, and plentiful use of emollients. Asteatotic eczema will often resolve with this approach. Additionally, venous eczema is helped by treating underlying venous insufficiency with leg elevation, support hosiery, or varicose vein surgery when appropriate.

Comparative features		
Disorder	**Asteatotic eczema**	**Venous eczema**
Age	Usually elderly	
Sex	Either	Female preponderance
Family history	Non-specific	There may be a history of venous disease, e.g. varicose veins, venous thrombosis, thrombophlebitis, or injury.
Sites	Typically, lower leg. If asteatosis is more extensive, or particularly severe, consider systemic causes (e.g. hypothyroidism, lymphoma or other malignancy) or other diagnoses (e.g. scabies).	Lower leg, especially above medial malleolus at the site of the lowest perforating vein connecting the superficial and deep venous systems. Scattered patches of eczema may occur at other sites (known as a secondary or 'autosensitization' eczema) if the venous eczema is particularly severe, complicated by a contact allergy, or infected.
Symptoms	None, itch–usually fairly abrupt onset	Itch–usually gradual onset
Signs common to both	Eczematous rash affecting lower legs; dry scaly erythematous rash	
Discriminatory signs	Symmetrical. Usually affects the anterior shin only. Typical 'crazy paving' morphology or parallel fissuring, and fine scale. There may be some purpuric spots within the fissures, especially if severe (e.g. acute onset paraneoplastic type) or if the patient is taking anticoagulants.	One or both legs are involved. Affects skin above medial malleolus mainly. Usually accompanied by other signs of venous disease (oedema, ulceration, venous flares, pigmentation, atrophy blanche, lipodermatosclerosis, Fig. 69.3)
Associated features	Areas of dry or scaly skin at other sites are common.	May be associated varicose veins, history of previous thrombosis, or leg ulceration. Mixed arterial and venous disease is common.
Important tests	None is usually required if there is an obvious explanation (e.g. frequent washing in a hospital environment). Consider systemic malignancy, nutritional deficiencies, if the extent or severity is atypical.	Assessment of arterial and venous circulation (a) to identify surgically correctable venous pathology, and (b) to determine adequate arterial supply for use of compression bandages or hosiery (see Table on p. 138)

Further reading:
p. 76, p. 110, p. 132, p. 138, p. 150, p. 154.

References

Fenske NA, Lober CW. Structural and functional changes of normal aging skin. *J Am Acad Dermatol* 1986; **15**:571–85.

Goldman MP, Weiss RA, Bergan JJ. Diagnosis and treatment of varicose veins: a review. *J Am Acad Dermatol* 1994; **31**:393–413.

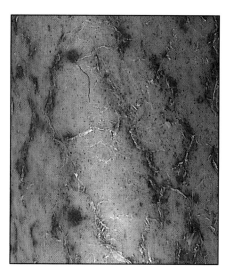

Figure 68.1
Asteatotic 'crazy paving' pattern of ichthyosis: the prominent purpuric component was due to thrombo-cytopaenia in this case.

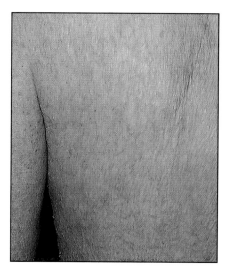

Figure 68.2
Asteatotic pattern on the trunk due to malignancy. As in Fig. 68.1, features such as unusual sites or severity suggest the possibility of underlying lymphoma or other internal malignancy.

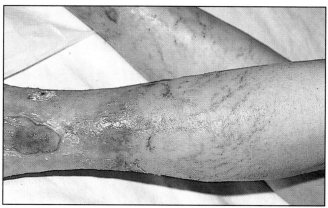

Figure 68.3 *Asteatotic eczema (proximal 'crazy-paving' pattern) in a patient with venous eczema and ulceration.*

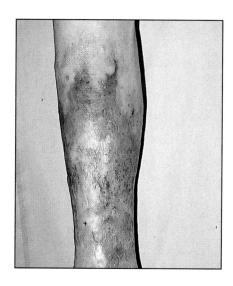

Figure 68.4 *Venous eczema with marked residual pigment-ation in a patient with obvious varicose veins.*

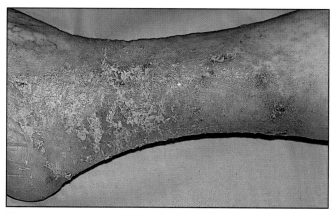

Figure 68.5 *Venous eczema and early ulceration: note that the changes are mainly on the medial aspect of the leg whereas asteatotic eczema is most prominent on the shins.*

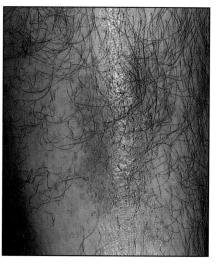

Figure 68.6
Schamberg's disease, showing a low-grade capillaritis causing haemosiderin deposition in the skin, in the absence of overt venous disease. Itch and ichthyotic skin (if they occur at all in this condition) are mild.

Common presenting feature: lower leg ulceration.

Rationale for comparison: treatment of these two types of ulceration is quite different when they occur in a pure form. However, in many patients, leg ulcers are the result of mixed arterial and venous disease and treatment of each component may aggravate the other. In particular, elevation and compression bandaging is the most important component of treatment for venous disease but will aggravate arterial symptoms.

Other differential diagnoses: vasculitis and inflammatory causes of leg ulceration (particularly pyoderma gangrenosum) (p. 140, Fig. 70.4); infective ulceration; necrobiosis lipoidica; ulcerated tumours.

Conclusion and key points: pure arterial ulcers are characteristically multiple, painful, punched-out, and situated on the shin and dorsum of the foot. The skin around them may be pale, erythematous, dusky or relatively normal in appearance, and there may be other symptoms and signs of arterial disease (claudication on walking or leg elevation, hair loss, or digital ischaemia). Venous ulcers are less commonly painful, arise mainly above the malleoli (especially medial) and have a background of venous damage (p. 136). The skin around a venous ulcer is pigmented, sclerotic, scarred (atrophie blanche), scaly or eczematous, and distended veins may be apparent on standing. Respective investigations and therapy differ, but in practice it is common for patients with venous disease to have some degree of associated arterial insufficiency.

Comparative features		
Disorder	**Arterial leg ulcer**	**Venous leg ulcer**
Age	Usually elderly	
Sex	Male predominance	Female predominance
Family history	Non-specific	There may be a personal or family history of venous disease.
Sites	Lower leg, especially shins, dorsal aspect of feet and digits	Lower leg, especially above medial malleolus
Symptoms	Pain, typically worsened by leg elevation (e.g. at night) and relieved by hanging the leg over the edge of a bed	May be painful, especially if infected
Signs common to both	Ulceration of lower leg	
Discriminatory signs	Usually multiple, with punched-out appearance. Surrounding skin may appear normal or ischaemic (pale, cool, mottled or dusky, with poor capillary refill and hair loss). There is usually bilateral evidence of arterial disease although not necessarily bilateral ulceration; if ulcers of arterial appearance are consistently unilateral, they may be due to cholesterol emboli from a discrete area of proximal atherosclerosis.	Usually solitary, affecting one or both legs. Typical sites are above the malleoli, especially medially. Ulcers occur on a background of venous disease including venous eczema, pigmentation, venous flare, varicose veins, scarring and sclerosis. Foot pulses are usually palpable unless there is oedema due to venous disease.
Associated features	Cigarette smoking, evidence of larger vessel disease (femoral or carotid bruits, loss of foot pulses), abdominal aortic aneurysm, etc. Toenail dystrophy may occur due to long-standing ischaemia.	Often associated with some degree of secondary lymphoedema
Important tests	Specialist investigations to demonstrate surgically correct proximal arterial stenoses, e.g. arteriography, duplex scan	Simple Doppler test of arterial pulses, because low pressures (ankle:brachial systolic pressure ratio less than 1.0) may preclude compression bandaging. Specialist tests to identify any surgically correctable venous disease

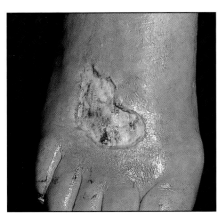

Figure 69.1 *Arterial ulcer, showing typical dorsal foot site and deep punched-out morphology. Note oedematous, erythematous, hairless, surrounding skin, without pigmentation or dermatitis.*

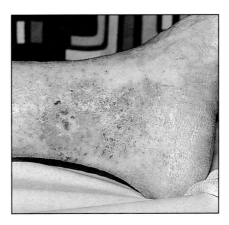

Figure 69.2 *Venous ulceration: there are several small areas of venous ulceration on a background of active stasis dermatitis.*

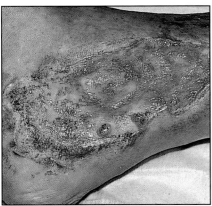

Figure 69.3 *Venous ulcer seen at typical medial malleolus site, and with adjacent pigmentation. The rather smooth, tight skin suggests an element of arterial compromise as well.*

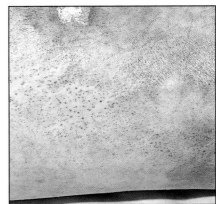

Figure 69.4. *Atrophie blanche: this is a feature of venous disease.*

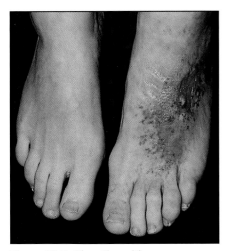

Figure 69.5 *Ulceration with some venous features at an unusual site, without any contralateral changes of venous stasis. This lesion was due to an arteriovenous malformation. Note the different-sized feet.*

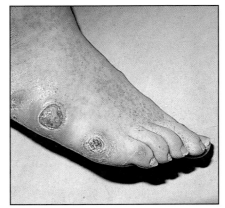

Figure 69.6 *Neuropathic ulcers: these have a similar punched-out appearance to arterial ulcers, but usually occur over bony prominences on the foot and are relatively asymptomatic. Underlying osteomyelitis should be excluded.*

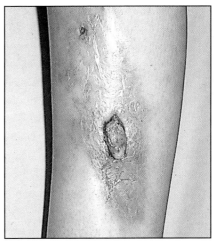

Figure 69.7 *Necrobiosis lipoidica in a diabetic patient: ulceration is often difficult to treat as the adjacent skin is atrophic and fragile.*

Further reading:
p. 136, pp. 140–144, p. 166.

References
Goldman MP, Weiss RA, Bergan JJ. Diagnosis and treatment of varicose veins: a review. *J Am Acad Dermatol* 1994; **31**:393–413.
Lowitt MH, Dover JS. Necrobiosis lipoidica. *J Am Acad Dermatol* 1991; **25**:735–48.

Phillips TJ, Dover JS. Leg ulcers. *J Am Acad Dermatol* 1991; **25**:965–87.
Ryan TJ. *The management of leg ulcers, 2nd edn.* Oxford University Press, Oxford, 1987.

Common presenting feature: lower leg ulceration.

Rationale for comparison: unlike venous ulcers, vasculitic ulcers require evaluation for systemic causes (including drug-induced vasculitis) and internal organ involvement, and usually need systemic therapy.

Other differential diagnoses: pyoderma gangrenosum; embolic ulceration; primary infections; papular urticaria (p. 142); ulcerated neoplasms.

Conclusion and key points: vasculitic ulcers are usually multiple and occur with other vasculitic lesions such as palpable purpura. However, some inflammatory types of ulceration, such as pyoderma gangrenosum, are usually solitary lesions without other skin signs at other sites. Confusion may occur as vasculitic ulceration often develops in the same region of the leg as venous ulcers, and may therefore occur with signs of venous disease (p. 136–138). This probably happens because the main site of immune-complex deposition in vasculitis is in the venules, which may already be damaged by venous insufficiency at this site. Confusion between the two disorders also occurs because purpura and haemosiderin deposition, though usually more apparent in vasculitis, are also features of venous eczema. Development of ulceration at the same time as crops of smaller lesions favours a diagnosis of vasculitis, and vasculitic ulcers generally enlarge faster, and crust or bleed more than venous ulcers.

Comparative features		
Disorder	**Venous leg ulcer**	**Vasculitic ulceration**
Age	Usually elderly	Any. The risk of vasculitic lesion ulceration increases with age.
Sex	Either	
Family history	May be positive for varicose veins but this is a poor discriminator	Non-specific
Sites	Lower leg, especially above medial malleolus	Vasculitis is usually most apparent on lower legs, but any body site may be affected (for example, buttocks in Henoch–Schonlein purpura). Ulceration occurring within areas of vasculitis is most frequent on digits or on the lower leg.
Symptoms	None, pain. Ulceration usually occurs as a gradual process unless it is provoked by an injury.	Usually painful and of sudden onset, often with purpuric papules for a day or two prior to development of larger ulcerated lesions
Signs common to both	Lower leg ulceration. Evidence of venous disease or oedema does not exclude vasculitis, as this is most likely to cause ulceration in older patients with pre-existing vascular disease.	
Discriminatory signs	Usually solitary/few. May have surface slough but not usually a hard crust. Always associated with other signs of venous disease.	Usually multiple lesions, which often appear in crops. Ulcers are typically accompanied by other vasculitic lesions such as palpable purpura, retiform (reticulate) purpura, digital infarcts or splinter haemorrhages.
Associated features	If purpura is present, it is usually within the distribution of venous eczema and does not form palpable lesions. Other evidence of venous disease is always present (pp. 136–138).	Vasculitis at other sites, e.g. buttocks, digits. Evidence of systemic disease caused by the vasculitis (e.g. renal involvement, arthropathy) or of an underlying systemic cause (e.g. rheumatoid arthritis)
Important tests	Assess arterial supply as discussed in p. 138	General medical and drug history for potential causes. Skin biopsy (histology and direct immunofluorescence), renal function, haematology, immunoglobulins, complement, collagen-vascular disease screen (ANA, ANCA etc), infection screen, depending on clinical pattern

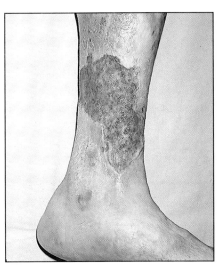

Figure 70.1 *Venous ulcer, showing typical site and adjacent pigmentation.*

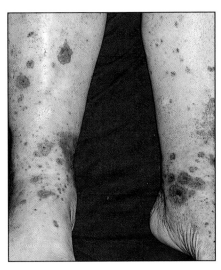

Figure 70.2. *Vasculitic ulceration with extensive palpable purpura in leukocytoclastic vasculitis.*

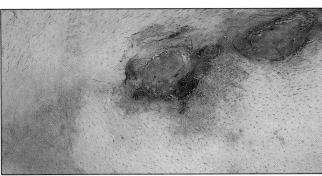

Figure 70.3 *Deeper ulceration within an area of livedo, in a patient with antiphospholipid syndrome.*

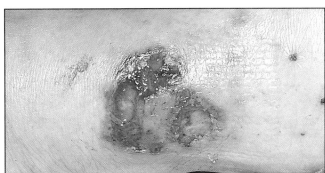

Figure 70.4 *Pyoderma gangrenosum: typical ragged ulcer with blue border. The major causes are inflammatory bowel disease, haematological malignancy and inflammatory joint disease.*

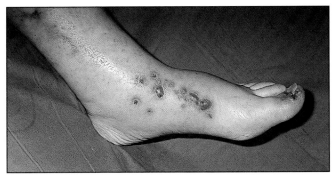

Figure 70.5 *Embolic vasculitis due to cholesterol emboli, in a patient with large vessel arteriosclerosis. This may mimic ischaemic arterial ulceration if there are few lesions, or may be more overtly vasculitic as in this case.*

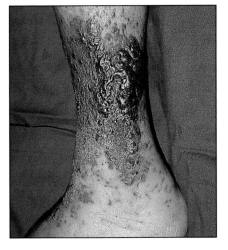

Figure 70.6 *Ulcerated tumours: these may mimic venous leg ulcers or vasculitis (see also p. 136). In this case, the lesion was an angiosarcoma.*

Further reading:
p. 136, p. 138, p. 142, p. 144, p. 166.

References
Ansell BM, Bacon PA, Lie JT, Yazici H. The vasculitides. *In Science and practice*. Chapman & Hall, London, 1996.
Powell FC, Su WPD, Perry HO. Pyoderma gangrenosum: classification and management. *J Am Acad Dermatol* 1996; **34**:395–409.
Ramsay C, Fry L. Allergic vasculitis. Clinical and histological features and incidence of renal involvement. *Br J Dermatol* 1969; **81**:96–102.
Sams WM, *et al*. Leukocytoclastic vasculitis. *Arch Dermatol* 1976; **112**:219–26.

Common presenting feature: itchy plaques and blisters on the lower leg.

Rationale for comparison: management of these two disorders is fundamentally different. Papular urticaria is due to insect bites and can often be prevented by environmental measures, e.g. eradicating fleas from pets and the household. Bullous pemphigoid is a potentially severe disorder which requires high-dose systemic corticosteroid therapy.

Other differential diagnoses: oedema blisters (p. 144, Fig. 72.3); drug eruptions (especially fixed drug eruptions); contact dermatitis (including plants); diabetic bullae.

Conclusion and key points: papular urticaria is a disorder of bullous and urticated insect-bite reactions. It predominantly occurs in children and young adults, but causes diagnostic problems in older patients in whom leg blisters are more often caused by bullous pemphigoid, eczema, oedema or drug reactions. Papular urticaria occurs mainly on exposed skin of the lower limbs above the level of the shoes and socks, but may be more widespread if a pet with fleas is allowed to sit on the owner's knees or sleep on beds, in children if they lie on the floor, or where the causative insect is encountered outside in gardens or fields. By contrast, lesions of bullous pemphigoid are typically much more widely distributed, although they can be limited to feet and lower legs. Blisters in papular urticaria (particularly due to flea-bites) may be grouped together. Contact and photocontact reactions to plants also commonly affect exposed skin but have a streaky linear distribution and may exhibit marked post-inflammatory pigmentation.

Comparative features		
Disorder	**Bullous pemphigoid**	**Papular urticaria**
Age	Mostly >70 yr	Any, but mainly children or young adults
Sex	Female predominance	Either
Family history	Non-specific	Other family members may be affected, but a negative family history does not exclude infestation of household pets, as not everyone will react to insect bites.
Sites	Any site, but blisters are often first apparent on lower limbs.	Mainly legs, but can be more widespread. Usually occurs on exposed skin of legs, depending on type of insect implicated (e.g. flea bites are typically above ankles, whereas mosquito bites affect any exposed skin).
Symptoms	Usually severe itch	
Signs common to both	Papules, urticated plaques, clear unilocular blisters (may be haemorrhagic). In isolation, the blisters in these two disorders may be indistinguishable clinically.	
Discriminatory signs	There is usually a preceding 'urticated' eczematous phase. Blistering usually progresses fairly rapidly to become widespread. Blisters may be up to 5 cm and several may arise on the same area of background erythema. Milia may occur at sites of healed lesions. Oral lesions occur in 5% of cases, and palmar pompholyx in 25%.	Lesions may show some grouping and tend to occur in crops. Blisters are fewer in number compared with pemphigoid, rarely larger than 2 cm in diameter, and more discrete, and occur without an eczematous background (although there are often some 'urticated' papular lesions). A central punctum may be visible, and healing may leave hyper-pigmented scars. No oral or palmar lesions occur.
Associated features	None	May be seasonal or related to specific exposure, e.g. visiting a household with a cat, gardening
Important tests	Biopsy for histology and immunofluorescence; baseline monitoring for systemic steroid therapy	Biopsy if uncertain. Demonstration of ectoparasites on pets by microscopy of coat brushings
Treatment	High-dose oral corticosteroids, immunosuppressive agents	Identify likely source. If appropriate, treat household pets and their environment. Use insect repellants, topical steroid to lesions

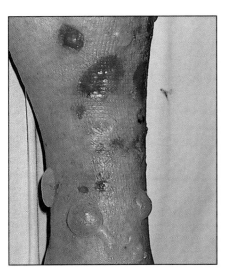

Figure 71.1 *Bullous pemphigoid: there are tense blisters and some erosions. In this case, the lesions have no background inflammation and papular urticaria would be a very reasonable differential diagnosis.*

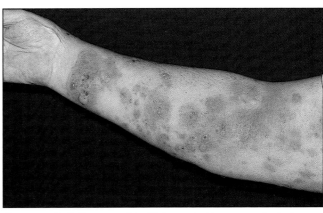

Figure 71.2 *Bullous pemphigoid demonstrating a more typical markedly 'urticated' background and some tense clear unilocular blisters.*

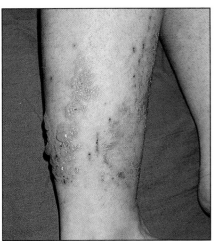

Figure 71.3 *Intensely bullous but very linear eruption: this is probably a plant contact dermatitis.*

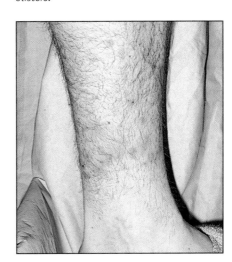

Figure 71.4 *Papular flea-bite reactions at a typical site around the top of the sock: note the typical grouping of lesions.*

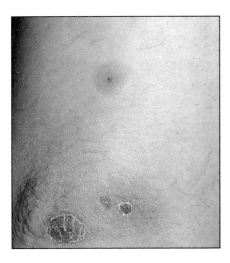

Figure 71.5 *Insect-bite reactions: these may have purpuric spots in the centre (known as purpura pulicosa). This is particularly prominent in this case which was caused by bedbug bites.*

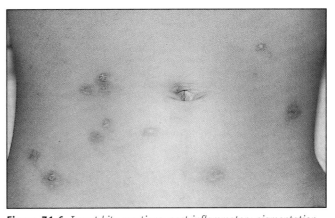

Figure 71.6 *Insect-bite reactions: post-inflammatory pigmentation of the skin is relatively common following insect-bite reactions, as shown here.*

Further reading:
p. 66, p. 94, p. 108, pp. 112–116, p. 144.

References
Burns DA. The investigation and management of arthropod bite reactions in the home. *Clin Exp Dermatol* 1987; **12**:114–20.

Charlesworth EN, Johnson JL. An epidemic of canine scabies in man. *Arch Dermatol* 1974; **110**:572–4.

Hewitt M, *et al*. Pet animal infestations and human skin lesions. *Br J Dermatol* 1971; **85**:215–25.

Common presenting feature: blisters on lower legs in elderly patients.

Rationale for comparison: these two conditions both occur primarily in elderly patients and are commonly confused. Incorrect diagnosis of oedema blisters as bullous pemphigoid may lead to unnecessary treatment with high-dose systemic corticosteroids.

Other differential diagnoses: papular urticaria (p. 142); contact allergy (including plants, Fig. 71.3); blisters in lymphoedema; diabetic bullosis; drug-induced bullae.

Conclusion and key points: oedema blisters usually occur in patients with obvious severe leg oedema, but sometimes appear to be related to the speed of development of oedema rather than its actual degree. They are most common in elderly patients with atrophic skin, particularly those who develop oedema suddenly as a result of stopping diuretics, such as before an operation or because of illness. Although oedema blisters are unilocular, as in pemphigoid, and occasionally haemorrhagic due to fragile skin, they do not arise on an inflammatory base and their fluid content is essentially colourless transudate, rather than the straw-coloured exudate typical of pemphigoid. They are usually asymptomatic, and unlike blisters of bullous pemphigoid they do not itch. Burst blisters may be sore due to exposure of the eroded dermis.

Comparative features		
Disorder	**Bullous pemphigoid**	**Oedema blister**
Age	Elderly	
Sex	Either, female predominance	Either
Family history	Non-specific	
Sites	Any; often initially affects legs	Lower legs
Symptoms	Itch, soreness	None, soreness if epithelium removed
Signs common to both	Unilocular blisters on lower leg(s)	
Discriminatory signs	Straw-coloured blister contents. Blisters usually arise on an urticated or eczematous background but some may develop on a non-inflamed base. Blisters are usually widely distributed on the leg and at other sites, and progressively increase in extent. Milia may occur in healed lesions.	Colourless blister fluid. Blisters all arise on non-inflamed base.
Associated features	Mouth lesions in 5% of cases, palmar pompholyx in 25%	Oedema of lower leg, typically increasing due to cardiac failure, discontinued diuretic therapy or other medical reasons (e.g. nephrotic syndrome)
Important tests	Biopsy for histology, immunofluorescence	As determined by underlying cardiac failure etc. Biopsy is not required, and is best avoided due to the risk of poor healing.

Further reading:
p. 114, p. 116, p. 142, p. 146.

References
Bork K. Cutaneous side-effects of drugs. WB Saunders, Philadelphia, 1988:113–14.
Cantwell AR, Martz W. Idiopathic bullae in diabetes. *Arch Dermatol* 1967; **96**:42–4.

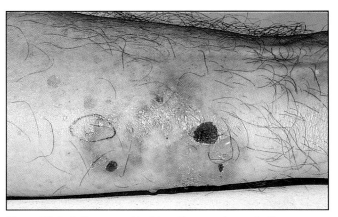

Figure 72.1 *Bullous pemphigoid on the arm, demonstrating 'urticated' lesions (see also p. 142) as well as blisters.*

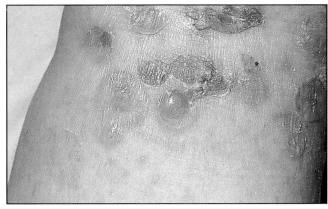

Figure 72.2 *Bullous pemphigoid, showing a less inflammatory form, which was localised to the foot. The blisters are more numerous and discrete than is typical of oedema blisters.*

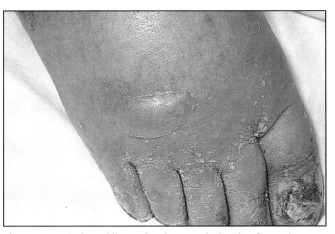

Figure 72.3 *Oedema blister, showing a typical rather featureless unilocular blister on an oedematous foot.*

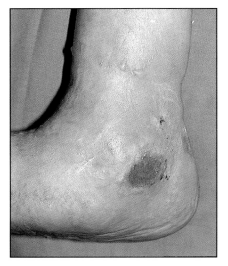

Figure 72.4 *Oedema blisters: there are smaller and more scattered blisters above the level of a recently removed bandage.*

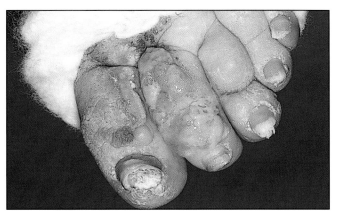

Figure 72.5 *Lymphoedema of the toes in a patient with chronic venous ulceration. The oedematous papules in this disorder may be confused with blisters as occurred in this case.*

Some drugs which cause bullae
Barbiturates   **Sulphonamides**   **Halides**   **Anticoagulants**   **Drug-induced pemphigus (captopril, penicillamine)**   **Pseudo-porphyria (frusemide, nalidixic acid, naproxen)**

Common presenting feature: swelling and tenderness of the lower leg.

Rationale for comparison: lower leg cellulitis is a disorder with significant long-term morbidity, so prompt and vigorous treatment is required. Similar appearances may occur due to deep venous thrombosis, or bilaterally due to acute or chronic oedema. These, and the other differential diagnoses listed, require different treatments and have different long-term significances, so distinction between them is important.

Other differential diagnoses: deep venous thrombosis; acute oedema (due to cardiac failure, hypoproteinaemia etc.); lymphoedema; venous eczema; tibial compartment syndrome; gout and acute musculoskeletal conditions; early herpes zoster; erythema nodosum and other panniculitides; erythema nodosum migrans.

Conclusion and key points: ascending cellulitis of the lower leg is usually due to streptococcal, or sometimes staphylococcal, infection. It is almost always unilateral and typically starts in the foot. However, initial symptoms may be in the calf. The commonest portal of entry, which is a useful pointer to the diagnosis, is toeweb maceration due to tinea pedis. Fever and systemic malaise are usually marked and, when present, differentiate cellulitis from most other differential diagnoses. In the elderly obese or chronically oedematous leg, or after a rapid increase in oedema, there may be significant erythema; this is a common source of diagnostic confusion. Cellulitis secondary to preceding venous eczema should be differentiated, as the commonest infection in such cases is staphylococcal. Similarly, cellulitis secondary to leg ulceration may be caused by a large variety of organisms including streptococci, staphylococci, *Pseudomonas* spp., *Bacteroides* spp., and others. Erythema nodosum is usually bilateral and the lesions are discrete, deep, tender erythematous nodules, but may be asymmetrical. Erythema nodosum migrans is morphologically similar, but is unilateral and more persistent.

Comparative features		
Disorder	**Lower leg cellulitis**	**Other causes of leg swelling**
Age	Any adult, but most frequently the elderly	
Sex	Minor female predominance	Either
Family history	May be positive	Non-specific
Sites	Rapid ascent up lower leg, usually initially with swelling and tenderness of dorsum of foot; may commence in calf	Usually first apparent at ankle
Symptoms	Local tenderness, systemic fever and malaise	None, sensation of tightness or pain (depending on cause and rate of evolution)
Signs common to both	Swelling and erythema of lower leg	
Discriminatory signs	Rapid ascent of erythema up the leg, usually confluent but sometimes with spared 'skip' lesions. Unilateral. Commonly tinea pedis is also present. Fever and malaise are typical; lymphangitis and tender lymphadenopathy are also common.	Simple oedema is not usually erythematous. In some individuals with obese or lymphoedematous legs, erythema may be prominent but is usually symmetrical.
Associated features	Chronic lymphoedema is both a predisposing factor and a consequence of recurrent episodes. Ulceration may occur.	Depends on cause. May be heart failure, pulmonary emboli etc.
Important tests	Bacteriology swabs if any blister or portal of entry. Mycology samples from tinea pedis. Serology (ASO titre) for streptococci	Depends on likely cause. May require ECG, chest X-ray, doppler, venography etc.

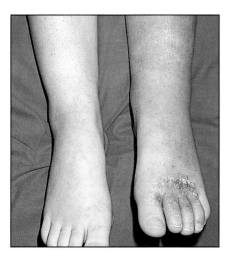

Figure 73.1
Resolving cellulitis of the leg in a patient with tinea pedis: fungal infection of the foot is the most frequent portal of entry for the causative streptococci.

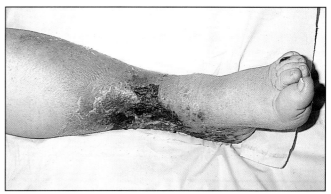

Figure 73.2 *Streptococcal cellulitis with secondary skin ulceration. In this case, the portal of entry was probably a foot callosity which had recently been pared. This may be confused with vasculitis.*

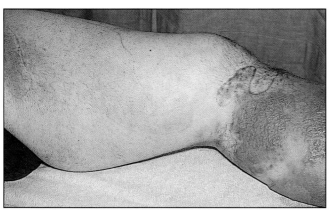

Figure 73.3. *Acute cellulitis demonstrating skip lesions, resembling vasculitis. The inked margin on the thigh demonstrates clearing with treatment.*

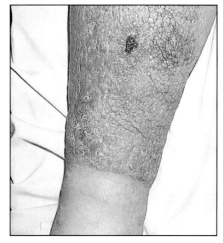

Figure 73.4
Lymphoedema: this is a condition which may be confused with cellulitis. This is not due to infection but it is important to treat any infection within lymphoedema aggressively to prevent deterioration.

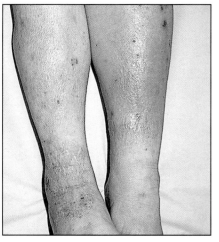

Figure 73.5 *Acute increase in chronic oedema of cardiac origin may produce both erythema and swelling, and may be confused with cellulitis but is usually symmetrical. Bilateral concurrent cellulitis is extremely uncommon.*

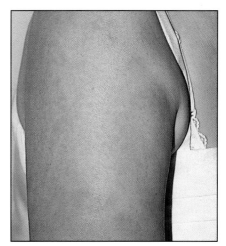

Figure 73.6 *Acute inflammatory connective tissue disorders, in this case a condition known as eosinophilic fasciitis, may mimic an infective cellulitis.*

Further reading:
p. 42, p. 136, pp. 140–144, p. 168.

References
Bernard P, *et al.* Streptococcal cause of erysipelas and cellulitis in adults. *Arch Dermatol* 1989; **125**:779–82.
Hannuksela M. Erythema nodosum migrans. *Acta Dermatovenereol* (Stockh) 1973; **53**:313–7.
Sachs MK. Cutaneous cellulitis. *Arch Dermatol* 1991; **127**:493–6.
Stevens DL. Invasive group A streptococcal infections. *Clin Infect Dis* 1992; **14**:2–13.

Common presenting feature: cold, discolored digits, usually fingers.

Rationale for comparison: Raynaud's phenomenon may be related to an underlying collagen vascular disorder or to another systemic cause. By comparison, acrocyanosis has no significant associations in the typical young age-group in which it occurs.

Other differential diagnoses: other connective tissue disease causing cold digits but without necessarily causing Raynaud's phenomenon, especially the chilblain variant of lupus erythematosus; neuropathies (e.g. carpal tunnel syndrome).

Conclusion and key points: Raynaud's phenomenon is an episodic vasoconstrictive process which affects one or few digits with a characteristic sharply demarcated blanching followed by vasodilation. It may be accompanied by signs of collagen vascular disorders, such as ragged cuticles, abnormal nailfold vasculature, sclerodactyly, splinter haemorrhages, and digital pulp infarcts. Raynaud's phenomenon may occur in the absence of any apparent underlying cause (usually in young women), may have local causes such as cervical rib (a cause of unilateral symptoms), or may be a feature of connective tissue disorders such as scleroderma (p. 44).

Acrocyanosis is a more gradual and predictable process which causes dusky discoloration or pallor of all digits simultaneously. The affected areas change colour to a redder or purple shade in warmer conditions, but still feel cool to the touch. Acrocyanosis may be accompanied by chilblains or by erythrocyanosis (a dusky cyanotic discoloration over fatty areas of the thigh or upper arms). Onset in children or young adults is rarely associated with any underlying cause, but onset in older patients may occur due to cryoglobulinaemia.

Comparative features		
Disorder	**Raynaud's phenomenon**	**Acrocyanosis/chilblains**
Age	Onset is usually in teens or young adulthood. Onset in middle-age or later is usually associated with an underlying systemic cause.	May occur in children but most patients present in young adult age-group
Sex	Marked female predominance (about 8:1 F:M)	Female predominance
Family history	May be positive	Non-specific
Sites	Digits, usually distal to proximal interphalangeal joint, variable and asymmetrical at any one time.	Acrocyanosis affects the entire hand or foot but is most marked in distal fingers or toes. All digits are affected symmetrically. Chilblains occur on digits, or as panniculitis of fatty areas (upper arms or thighs).
Symptoms	Episodic white, cold, clumsy fingers, with subsequent burning and erythema, affecting one or several digits	Cold clumsy digits, pain on rewarming. Persistent itch or burning pain of chilblains when the skin is warm
Signs common to both	Pallor and cyanosis of digits precipitated by cold	
Discriminatory signs	Sharp proximal demarcation of pallor affecting one or a few digits only	General, symmetrical, dusky discoloration of digits and remainder of hand, which always feels cold to the touch
Associated features	There may be signs of an associated collagen vascular disease (see figures). Nailfold telangiectasia, sclerodactyly and nail ridges may occur in severe Raynaud's even in cases with no identifiable cause.	Acrocyanosis may be associated with erythrocyanosis (dusky cold areas of skin on thighs, calves or upper arms) or prominent physiological livedo causing reticulate mottling of cool fatty areas. Chilblains may occur either at sites of acrocyanosis or over fatty areas.
Important tests	Serology for collagen vascular disease, other tests if clinically indicated (e.g. if confined to one hand, consider thoracic outlet disorders such as cervical rib)	Consider medical causes (e.g. hypothyroidism, myelo-proliferative disorders) if later age of onset. Exclude a cold-precipitating protein, especially cryoglobulinaemia, if severe and/or progressive or if other features such as vasculitis are present.

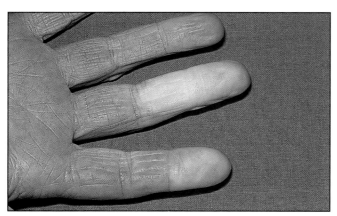

Figure 74.1 *Raynaud's phenomenon, showing isolated transient digital ischaemia.*

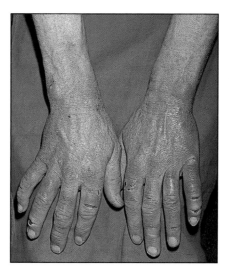

Figure 74.2
Severe acrocyanosis with digital chilblains. Note the symmetry, plus the involvement of digits and the hands.

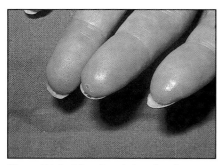

Figure 74.3 *Sclerodactyly in scleroderma, showing tight skin and small pulp infarct.*

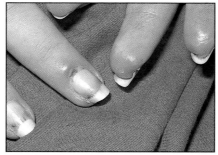

Figure 74.4 *Digital infarcts and splinter haemorrhages in acute scleroderma. The patient had a history of severe Raynaud's phenomenon.*

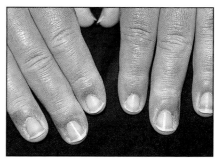

Figure 74.5 *Nailfold oedema and dusky erythema in systemic lupus erythematosus, which is another cause of Raynaud's phenomenon.*

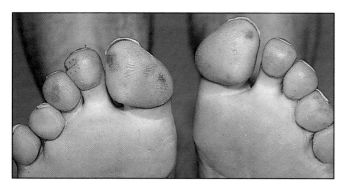

Figure 74.6 *Digital chilblains: these are a common cause of diagnostic problems as they may appear very vasculitic.*

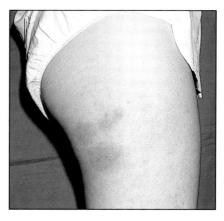

Figure 74.7
Equestrian panniculitis: this is a variant of chilblains which occurs on lateral thighs, typically in horse riders or others exposed to cold wet weather, and tight clothing or friction.

Further reading:
p. 6, p. 44.

References
Cox NH. Out in the cold: low temperature dermatology. *Dermatol Pract* 1994; **2**:9–11.
Doutre MS, *et al*. Chilblain lupus erythematosus: report of 15 cases. *Dermatology* 1992; **184**:26–8.

Su WP, *et al*. Chilblain lupus erythematosus (lupus pernio). Clinical review of Mayo clinic experience and proposal of diagnostic criteria. *Cutis* 1994; **54**:395–9.
Winterbauer RH. Multiple telangiectases, Raynaud's phenomenon, sclerodactyly and subcutaneous calcinosis. *Bull Johns Hopkins Hosp* 1964; **114**:361–83.

Common presenting feature: itchy thickened areas of skin on shins.

Rationale for comparison: lichen simplex is caused by chronic rubbing and, though it may recur, usually responds to antipruritic treatments (e.g. topical corticosteroids) with occlusive bandaging. Lichen planus (LP) is less responsive to treatment, particularly on lower legs and the two disorders therefore have different prognoses.

Other differential diagnoses: eczemas (discoid, asteatotic and venous); lichenoid drug eruptions; nodular prurigo; persistent insect-bite reactions; lichen amyloidosis.

Conclusion and key points: LP on the shins is often hypertrophic and not recognized as it may look different, and is usually more chronic, compared to LP at other sites. However, like LP at other sites, it generally has a purplish colour and post-inflammatory pigmentation. Oral lesions (striae on the buccal mucosa, Fig. 8.1) are common in typical lichen planus but less consistently present when it is essentially localized to the shins. Hypertrophic LP usually requires strong topical corticosteroid therapy. The commonest misdiagnosis is lichen simplex which is more linear due to chronic rubbing of the itchy area, and characteristically has accentuation of the skin surface ridges (lichenification). This condition often responds well to topical corticosteroids combined with occlusive bandaging, though there is a tendency to recurrence.

Comparative features		
Disorder	**Lichen simplex**	**Lichen planus (LP)**
Age	Usually young adult	Any; localized lower leg lesions are most common in the 40–60 yr age-group.
Sex	Either, with some site differences. Lichen simplex on legs and feet is more common in men, while lesions on the neck are more common in women.	Either
Family history	Non-specific; may be atopic tendency	Rarely positive
Sites	Shin, upper outer calf or dorsum/instep of foot. Other sites which may be affected include nape of neck, dorsal forearm, scrotum, vulva, sacrum, palms.	Anterolateral lower leg. Other common sites, which may coexist but where lesions are usually less verrucous, include the flexor aspect of the wrists and the buccal mucosa.
Symptoms	Itch, may be severe	
Signs common to both	Lichenified plaques, variable excoriation, variable degree of pigmentation	
Discriminatory signs	Usually obvious prominence of skin markings (lichenification), rather cobblestoned papular surface, some scaling; usually less well demarcated than LP	Lesions are more sharply defined. Their surface is more verrucous at this body site, compared with LP at other sites. LP has a typical purplish colour and marked post-inflammatory pigmentation at sites of resolved lesions. Lesions may be annular, and localization to sites of minor injury (Koebner reaction) may occur. Classic Whickham's striae of LP may be difficult to see in lesions on legs, but are present in lesions at other body sites.
Associated features	There may be an underlying cause of itch, usually dry asteatotic skin or atopy.	LP at other sites is fairly common (but these may be resolved lesions, as lower legs are typically slow to respond). Oral lesions are less common than in patients with generalized LP.
Important tests	None	Usually none; may need biopsy confirmation. Consider drug-induced lichenoid reactions (beta-blockers, gold, thiazides, antimalarials). An association with hepatitis C has recently been reported. Its prevalence in the UK population is, however, unknown.

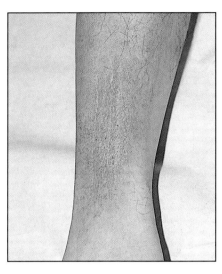

Figure 75.1 *Lichen simplex: the effect of recent scratching is clearly visible as linear accentuation of the surface scaling.*

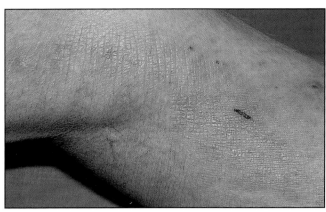

Figure 75.2 *Lichenification in an atopic: note the exaggerated skin creases and linear distribution due to scratching.*

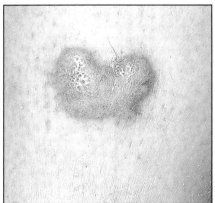

Figure 75.3 *Lichen planus on the leg, more nodular than at other body sites, but still with the characteristic purplish colour.*

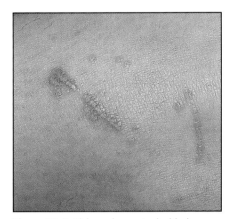

Figure 75.4 *Lichen planus: typical lesions demonstrating the Koebner reaction of localization to an area of minor scratch injury.*

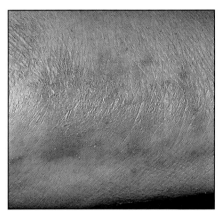

Figure 75.5 *Lichen planus, showing a flatter and more patchy lower leg lesion. Note the colour.*

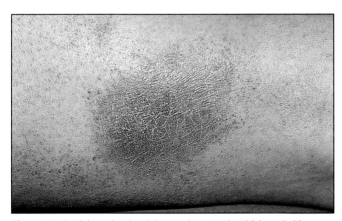

Figure 75.6 *Lichen simplex (close-up): note the thickened skin, exaggerated skin markings and pigmentation.*

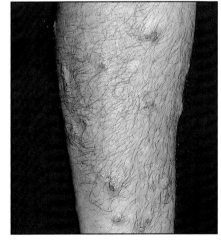

Figure 75.7 *Nodular prurigo: this shows a pattern of skin response in some patients with chronic itch of various causes. The nodules may resemble lichen planus of the legs, but the chronicity and behaviour of these is more suggestive of lichen simplex.*

Further reading:
p. 16, p. 102, p. 110, p. 132, p. 136, p. 154.

References
Boyd AS, Neldner KH. Lichen planus. *J Am Acad Dermatol* 1991; **25**:593–619.

Halevy S, Shai A. Lichenoid drug eruptions. *J Am Acad Dermatol* 1993; **29**:249–55.

Common presenting feature: pigmented skin lesion.

Rationale for comparison: dermatofibromas are one of the most frequently misdiagnosed localized skin lesions. They usually require no treatment, but if mistaken for an unusual naevus and excised, they often leave poor quality scars.

Other differential diagnoses: cysts; skin appendage neoplasms; giant comedones; melanoma; granulomas (e.g. post-vaccination, insect bite reaction, foreign body).

Conclusion and key points: dermatofibromas (pigmented histiocytomas) are frequently misdiagnosed and unnecessarily excised. They are much firmer than naevi, which are smooth and rubbery in texture, and can generally be easily differentiated from epidermoid cysts which are not pigmented and have no surface roughness. Dermatofibromas are tethered within the dermis, and can be palpated within the skin; they usually have marginal accentuation of pigmentation and surface roughness, neither of which are common features of naevi or cysts. Early dermatofibromas may be more vascular and itchy, but still have the characteristic firmness and tethering (dimple sign), and are unlikely to be confused with naevi.

Comparative features		
Disorder	**Naevus**	**Dermatofibroma**
Age	Most appear in teenage to young adult years	
Sex	Either	
Family history	Non-specific	
Sites	Any site, usually multiple	Mainly limbs, often a few lesions are present
Symptoms	Usually none	May itch in early stages, may be painful if traumatized
Signs common to both	Pigmented skin lesion	
Discriminatory signs	Usually uniform pigmentation, rubbery texture and normal surface without scaling	Marginal pigmentation. Surface roughness due to hyperkeratosis. Firm texture and tethering within the dermis (dimple sign)
Associated features	None	
Important tests	None	

Further reading:
p. 12, pp. 46–50, pp. 158–164.

References
Arnold HL, Tildon IL. Histiocytoma cutis. *Arch Dermatol* 1943; **47**:498–516.
Cerio R, Spaull J, Wilson Jones E. Dermatofibroma: a tumour of dermal dendrocytes? *J Cutan Pathol* 1987; **14**:351.

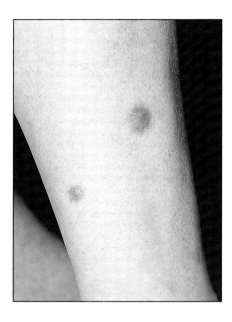

Figure 76.1 *Multiple dermatofibromas: these are relatively acute erythematous stage lesions.*

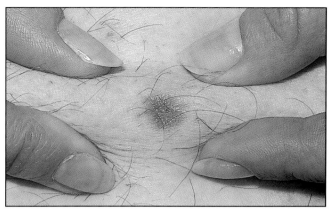

Figure 76.2 *Dermatofibroma: the 'dimple sign' due to dermal tethering is characteristic.*

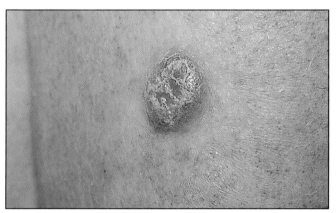

Figure 76.3 *Dermatofibroma: this is an older and more pigmented lesion. Surface roughness or scaling is common.*

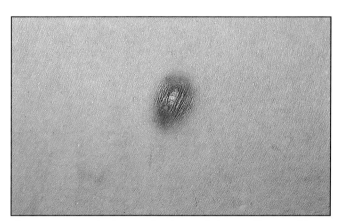

Figure 76.4 *Deeply pigmented and smooth dermatofibroma: this may resemble a blue naevus.*

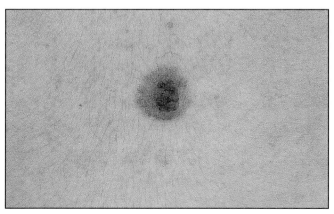

Figure 76.5 *Variably pigmented naevus with darker central colour. Dermatofibromas may also have a halo pattern of pigmentation, but usually have the darker pigment at the periphery.*

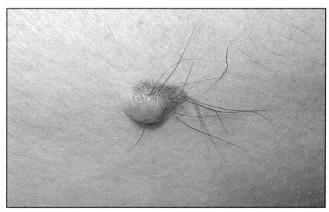

Figure 76.6 *Benign naevus: hair growth is a sign of a benign naevus, and is not a feature of dermatofibroma.*

Common presenting feature: hyperkeratotic skin lesions.

Rationale for comparison: porokeratosis is the term used for a characteristic morphology of skin lesions, in which the lesions are annular with an elevated scaly rim and an atrophic centre. Lesions of the commonest variety, known as disseminated superficial actinic porokeratosis (DSAP), are commonly confused with actinic keratoses as both occur in sun-damaged skin. However, the precise relationship to sunlight is less clear for DSAP.

Other differential diagnoses: seborrhoeic keratoses; Bowen's disease; squamous cell carcinoma; stucco keratoses; Kyrle's disease; Flegel's disease.

Conclusion and key points: disseminated superficial actinic porokeratosis (DSAP) is the most frequent form of porokeratosis and the most likely to be misdiagnosed. It occurs particularly in women and may be familial. Patients typically present at a younger age than patients with actinic keratoses. DSAP is morphologically striking and probably underdiagnosed. Other variants of porokeratosis include isolated larger lesions (Mibelli type) and linear types. Porokeratosis of all types generally responds poorly to treatment.

Comparative features		
Disorder	**Actinic keratosis**	**Porokeratosis**
Age	Mostly >60 yr	Most patients with DSAP are aged >50 yr; other types of porokeratosis may present in childhood.
Sex	Either: male predominance on limbs (mainly forearms)	Mainly female due to the predominance of women with DSAP
Family history	Non-specific	Occasionally positive
Sites	Mainly face and dorsum of hands; in males, frequently also affects scalp, ears and forearms	Mainly female lower leg
Symptoms	May be irritable, itchy	
Signs common to both	Hyperkeratotic lesions	
Discriminatory signs	Site distribution as above. Typically, spiky conical-shaped hyperkeratosis	Site distribution. Typically annular morphology with normal or slightly atrophic skin centrally
Associated features	Other signs of solar damage	Other signs of solar damage, but not usually as prominent as seen with actinic keratoses. The two disorders may coexist.
Important tests	Biopsy if fleshier base or hypertrophic (to exclude squamous cell carcinoma)	
Treatment	None required for minor lesions. Curettage, cryotherapy, excision, or 5-fluorouracil depending on the clinical situation	None usually required. Treatments as for actinic keratoses have all been used, but response is often poor.

Further reading:
p. 40, p. 52, p. 54, p. 56, p. 78, p. 156.

References
Chernosky ME, Freeman RG. Disseminated superficial actinic porokeratosis (DSAP). *Arch Dermatol* 1967; **96**:611–24.
Lucker GPH, Steijlen PM. The coexistence of linear and giant porokeratosis associated with Bowen's disease. *Dermatologica* 1994; **189**:78–80.

Rahberi H, Cordero AA, Mehregan AM. Linear porokeratosis: a distinctive clinical variant of porokeratosis of Mibelli. *Arch Dermatol* 1974; **109**:526–8.

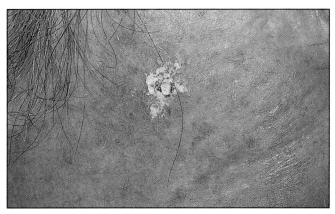

Figure 77.1 *Actinic keratosis on the face. The hard white spiky keratinization is typical.*

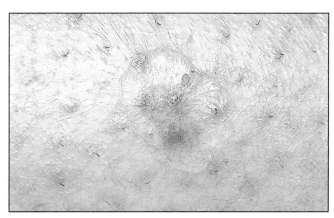

Figure 77.2 *Porokeratosis: close-up view to demonstrate the characteristic border and slight atrophy centrally.*

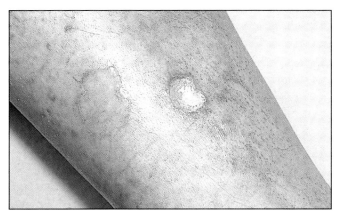

Figure 77.3 *Porokeratosis: lesions on the legs may become more keratotic as shown in the smaller of these two lesions.*

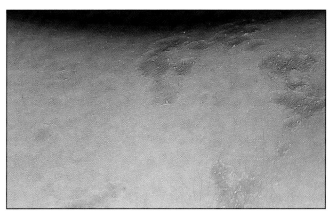

Figure 77.4 *Porokeratosis, showing more confluent and atrophic lesions.*

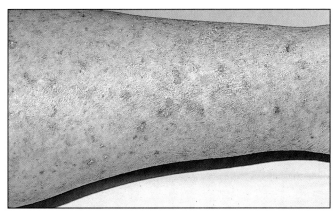

Figure 77.5 *Diffuse actinic keratoses in a relatively young patient with considerable previous solar and sunbed exposure (she had also had a squamous cell carcinoma of the inner thigh).*

Figure 77.6
Erythema ab igne: this is a disorder of infra-red damage to skin, in which keratoses may develop.

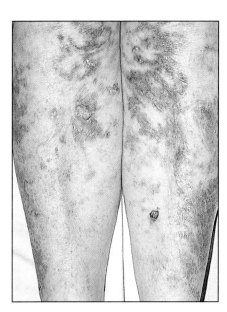

155

Common presenting feature: discrete scaling or crusted erythematous plaque(s).

Rationale for comparison: Bowen's disease is a superficial intraepidermal tumour which occurs mainly at sun-exposed sites. It can be successfully treated with various modalities. It is useful to differentiate it from more significant tumours, as well as from some benign dermatoses (p. 134), and it is important to be aware that invasive squamous cell carcinoma (SCC) may occur.

Other differential diagnoses: SCC (which may develop from lesions of Bowen's disease); basal cell carcinoma (BCC)(p. 86); porokeratosis (p. 154); clear cell acanthoma; seborrhoeic keratosis (p. 162); actinic keratosis (p. 40, p. 78, p. 154); other keratoses (e.g.

post-irradiation); some inflammatory dermatoses (especially discoid eczema, see Figs. 43.3, 51.3); venous eczema (p. 138); psoriasis (p. 102).

Conclusion and key points: Bowen's disease typically occurs on the lower leg of women in temperate climates, though facial lesions are more likely in sunnier climates. On both the leg and face, Bowen's disease forms radially expanding lesions for which the therapeutic problems are different compared with vertically invasive tumours. A firm diagnosis may therefore alter the approach to treatment. SCC may be difficult to differentiate from Bowen's disease, and often occurs on the leg. BCCs are relatively uncommon on the leg, but often look very different at this site compared with more typical facial lesions, and as a result are easily confused with Bowen's disease.

Comparative features		
Disorder	**Bowen's disease**	**Other skin malignancies**
Age	Adult, increases with age	
Sex	Female predominance in temperate climates	Either. Male predominance of squamous cell carcinoma (SCC)
Family history	Non-specific	Usually non-specific; sometimes positive, e.g. Gorlin's (naevoid basal cell carcinoma) syndrome, in which patients have multiple basal cell carcinomas, palmar pits, odontogenic cysts, bifid ribs, and other skeletal and neurological abnormalities
Sites	Usually occurs on the lower leg in temperate climates, and on head and neck in sunnier climates	Mostly on exposed sites, but up to 10% of basal cell carcinomas (BCC) are truncal. Diagnostic confusion is particularly likely on the lower leg due to the atypical appearance of BCC at this site.
Symptoms	Usually none	
Signs common to both	Localized erythematous scaly or crusted plaque(s)	
Discriminatory signs	Slow radial expansion. Irregular geographical outline. Crusted but not usually ulcerated or verrucous; if this is a feature it suggests SCC arising within a patch of Bowen's disease. Often multiple	SCC is more exophytic, crusted or verrucous. Keratoacanthoma (pp. 52–53) has more eruptive evolution, symmetrical shape, and a central horn. BCC usually has a smoother surface and more circular border. Clear cell acanthoma has a more shiny, moist red surface.
Associated features	There may be a history or clinical evidence of exposure to arsenic; this was still used in 'tonics' up to the 1950s, and may be suspected if palmar pits and keratoses are present (see Figs 43.6, 67.6)	
Important tests	Usually biopsy and excision. May not be necessary for small thin lesions in specialist departments	Biopsy and excision

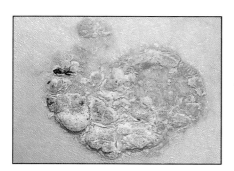

Figure 78.1 *Bowen's disease: note irregularity of crusting and geographical outline.*

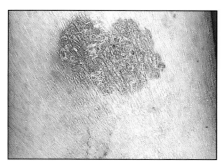

Figure 78.2 *Bowen's disease, showing a thin lesion at a typical lower leg site, again with geographical outline.*

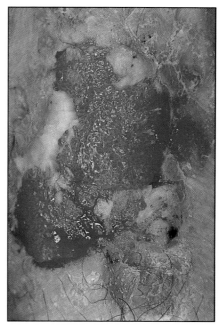

Figure 78.3 *Squamous cell carcinoma: this is a thicker and moister lesion with crusting.*

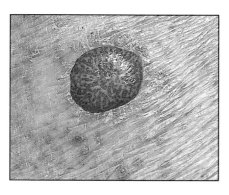

Figure 78.4 *Basal cell carcinoma: these look more moist and vascular than the same tumour at other sites, and are less easy to diagnose on clinical grounds.*

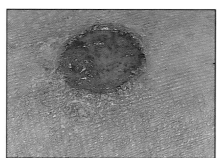

Figure 78.5 *Squamous cell carcinoma: this is an ulcerated lesion with a raised border.*

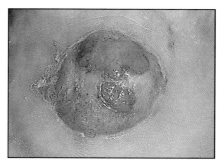

Figure 78.6 *Amelanotic melanoma on the heel: lesions of the foot in elderly patients raise a suspicion of this diagnosis, and absence of pigment is common at this site.*

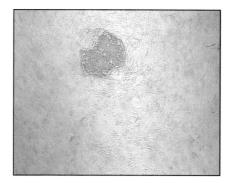

Figure 78.7 *Clear cell acanthoma: a benign tumour which is typically red and moist.*

Figure 78.8 *Seborrhoeic keratosis on the leg: these benign lesions may be less keratotic at this site compared with more typical truncal lesions (see also p. 56 and Fig. 67.5.)*

Further reading:
pp. 52–56, p. 78, p. 86, p. 98, p. 126, p. 128, p. 134, p. 154.

References
Cox NH. Body site distribution of Bowen's disease. *Br J Dermatol* 1994; **130**:714–6.
Kossard S, Rosen R. Cutaneous Bowen's disease. An analysis of 1001 cases. *J Am Acad Dermatol* 1992; **27**:406–10.

MacKie RM. *Skin cancer*, 2nd edn. Martin Dunitz, London, 1996.
Yeh S, How SH, Lin CS. Arsenical cancer of the skin. Histologic study with special reference to Bowen's disease. *Cancer* 1968; **21**:312–39.

Malignant melanoma v. angioma/pyogenic granuloma

Common presenting feature: deeply pigmented or bleeding skin lesion.

Rationale for comparison: angiomas, particularly if traumatized or infected, may be easily confused with melanoma. However, they require only local treatment whereas melanomas may require wide excision, histological staging, and prolonged follow-up. Any vascular lesion which is excised should be submitted for histological examination.

Other differential diagnoses: naevi (especially excoriated or with folliculitis); blue naevi; dermatofibroma; lymphangioma.

Conclusion and key points: thrombosis or bleeding within a previously red angioma, or bleeding into a clear vesicular lymphangioma, may cause a sudden colour change. This change may be sufficiently dark or black for it to be confused with melanin pigmentation. However, such changes in colour typically occur within 24–48 hours, and are therefore too rapid to suggest melanoma if an accurate history is obtainable. Very dark and slowly enlarging vascular lesions, such as venous lakes on the lips, may also cause diagnostic problems. The opposite problem rarely arises with rapidly growing poorly differentiated melanomas, which may be amelanotic (Fig. 78.6); these may present as non-pigmented vascular nodules and may therefore be misdiagnosed as more common eruptive vascular processes such as pyogenic granulomas. The latter typically occur on fingers (Figs 89.4 and 90.6), face (especially lips) and shoulder/upper arm; they should always be submitted for histological examination when removed.

Comparative features		
Disorder	**Malignant melanoma**	**Angioma**
Age	Any, very rare in childhood	Any. Pyogenic granuloma is rare in the elderly and amelanotic melanoma should be suspected.
Sex	Either, but female predominance	Either
Family history	May be positive for melanoma or atypical naevi	Non-specific
Sites	Any	Any. Most potential confusion with melanoma applies to: (i) angiomas which are subject to trauma or rubbing, e.g. waistline, or (ii) pyogenic granulomas, which typically occur on fingers, lips or face, or shoulder region
Symptoms	Usually none unless ulcerated. The history is of gradual growth rather than sudden change.	May be painful if injured or thrombosed; such changes usually occur within 24 h. Intermittent heavy bleeding
Signs common to both	Dark-coloured or bleeding skin lesion	
Discriminatory signs	Pigmentation is usually more varied than in angioma (colours include shades of brown, red, black, white, grey). The margin is irregular and asymmetrical. Bleeding and ulceration are late features. Unlike many angiomas, melanomas are not compressible.	Pigment is red or black (old bleeding) rather than brown, but haemosiderin deposition can be confusing. Usually sharp border, often compressible. Pyogenic granulomas enlarge rapidly, are moist or crusted, and bleed freely.
Associated features	There may be atypical naevi at other sites.	Usually none
Important tests	Excision and histology, clinical evaluation for lymphadenopathy and other tests depending on thickness and stage	Excision if diagnostic doubt or if bleeding, with histology (laser treatment or cautery are options if diagnosis is certain). Always exclude melanoma if angiomas arise at unusual sites or in the elderly.

Further reading:
p. 152, p. 160, p. 162, p. 180.

References
MacKie RM. *Skin cancer*, 2nd edn. Martin Dunitz, London, 1996.
Warner J, Wilson Jones E. Pyogenic granuloma recurring with multiple satellites. *Br J Dermatol* 1968; **80**:218–27.

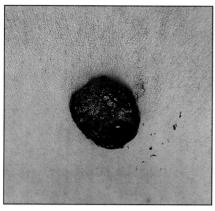

Figure 79.1 *Nodular melanoma: this is a very black, rapidly enlarging, lesion with surface bleeding.*

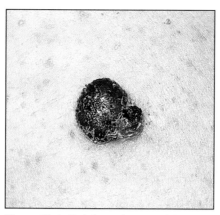

Figure 79.2 *Nodular melanoma with a more purple colour; this could easily be confused with an angioma or other vascular nodule.*

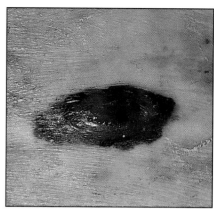

Figure 79.3 *Malignant melanoma: an ulcerated lesion with bleeding, but note the irregular margin and colour variation typical of a melanoma.*

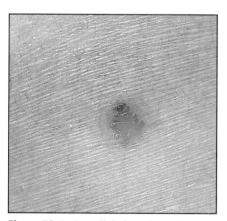

Figure 79.4 *A small dark angioma: this was referred as a pigmented lesion to exclude melanoma. The lobulated morphology is typical of an angioma.*

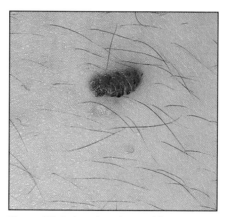

Figure 79.5 *Lymphangioma: this demonstrates the clear vesicular 'frog-spawn' appearance. Note the bleeding into the lower part of the lesion.*

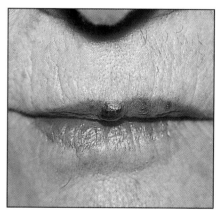

Figure 79.6 *Venous lake on the lip: these lesions may be confused with pigmented lentigines or melanoma, but are uniformly blue in colour and can be compressed.*

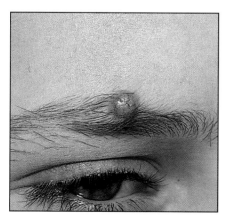

Figure 79.7 *Spitz naevus: this is an eruptive pattern of naevus, which typically occurs on the face in children. Clinically it appears vascular and the histological appearance may be suggestive of melanoma, but it is a benign melanocytic lesion.*

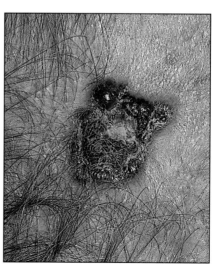

Figure 79.8
Pigmented basal cell carcinoma: these lesions are commonly confused with either melanoma or angioma. The pigment is usually dark grey or black, and arranged in coarse clumps within the lesion.

Common presenting feature: brown skin lesion.

Rationale for comparison: almost 50% of melanomas are believed to arise from pre-existing naevi. Early detection of malignant change should improve prognosis.

Other differential diagnoses: unusual but benign variants of melanocytic naevi (e.g. naevus 'en cocarde', 'dysplastic'/atypical naevi, palm/sole naevi); other changing melanocytic naevi (e.g. scratched naevi, naevi with episodes of folliculitis; halo naevi; Meyerson's [halo eczema] naevus); dermatofibroma; seborrhoeic keratoses.

Conclusion and key points: all naevi change during life. There is a gradual increase in numbers and size of naevi during childhood and early adult life in virtually all individuals; darkening of naevi is common in pregnancy and in summer months, and occasional trauma or folliculitis transiently alters the size and appearance of naevi. The main clue to determine malignancy is a progressive change in comparison with other previously similar naevi. Irregularity of edge or pigmentation, increasing size, itch and ulceration are all features which may support the diagnosis.

Comparative features		
Disorder	**Malignant melanoma**	**Naevus**
Age	Any, very rare in childhood	Most naevi appear before the age of 25 yr, especially during the 2nd decade.
Sex	Either, but female predominance	Either
Family history	May be positive for melanoma or atypical naevi	Inevitably positive. Young adult Caucasians in the UK have an average of 25 naevi.
Sites	Any	
Symptoms	Usually none but may itch. Ulceration or bleeding are late features.	Usually none but may itch (especially if scratched or due to an episode of folliculitis); may scab or bleed after trauma
Signs common to both	Variably pigmented skin lesion	
Discriminatory signs	A clear history of an individually changing lesion is the best discriminator in early melanoma. Increasing size, an irregular edge, and varied and asymmetrical pigmentation are characteristic. Ulceration is less common as it is a late feature, and occurs in lesions with other more typical changes also present.	Usually in context of several other naevi of similar colour. Many ordinary naevi have more than one shade of brown but black colours are uncommon, and varied colours if present are usually symmetrical about long and short axes. Change in elevation (increasing dome shape) is a common and normal maturation change in naevi.
Associated features	None specific, but large numbers or other clinically atypical naevi increase suspicion.	
Important tests	Excision and histology	Excision, referral, or document and review (photograph or measurement) if uncertainty
Other naevus variants	Malignancy is often a concern in naevi on palms, soles or scrotum but these do not have higher risk. However, palm and sole naevi are often somewhat atypical histologically, and melanoma of the foot has a poor prognosis which is probably due to late presentation.	Halo naevi (depigmented ring around a naevus, see Fig. 45.5) typically occur on the trunk in children, are usually multiple, and are benign. Meyerson's naevi have a discrete ring of surrounding eczema, with a central benign naevus. Spitz naevi are illustrated in Fig. 80.5.

Further reading:
p. 12, p. 46, p. 50, p. 56, p. 70, p. 152, p. 162, p. 180.

References
Halpern AC, *et al*. Dysplastic nevi as risk markers of sporadic (nonfamilial) melanoma. *Arch Dermatol* 1991; **129**:995–9.
Johnson TM, *et al*. Current therapy for malignant melanoma. *J Am Acad Dermatol* 1995; **32**:689–707.
Slade J, *et al*. Atypical mole syndrome: risk factor for cutaneous malignant melanoma and implications for management. *J Am Acad Dermatol* 1995; **32**:479–94.

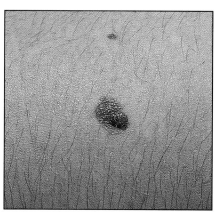

Figure 80.1 *A changing naevus with an eccentrically placed, elevated darker region in which the presumed diagnosis of melanoma was confirmed.*

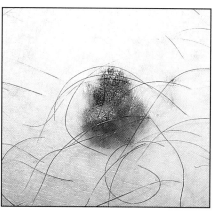

Figure 80.2 *Superficial spreading melanoma with a typical irregular asymmetrical margin, asymmetrical pigment variation, and a depigmented region.*

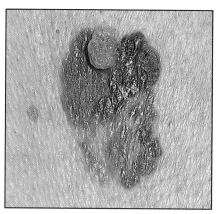

Figure 80.3 *Superficial melanoma: this is a more obvious superficial spreading melanoma on the back. The pink fleshy 'tag' is part of a pre-existing naevus.*

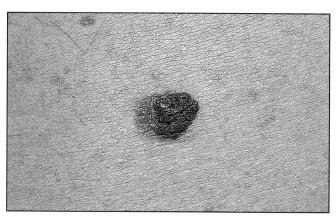

Figure 80.4 *Malignant melanoma, showing a relatively banal pale brown naevus but with an eccentrically situated darker brown raised area.*

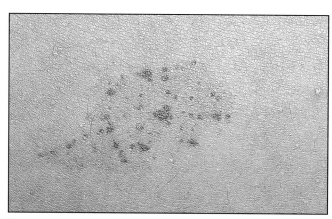

Figure 80.5 *Naevus spilus: this is a benign speckled lentiginous naevus. Melanoma in these lesions is extremely rare despite the unusual appearance.*

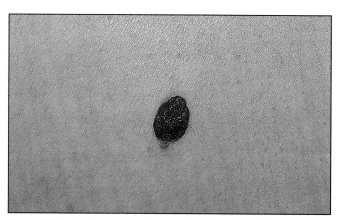

Figure 80.6 *Benign naevus: despite the dark colour, this naevus was unchanging and regular in morphology.*

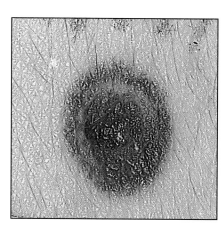

Figure 80.7 *Benign naevus, showing a benign pattern, with a rosette appearance known as an 'en cocarde' naevus.*

Common presenting feature: common pigmented skin lesions.

Rationale for comparison: seborrhoeic keratoses are benign. They are often either misdiagnosed or loosely described as 'moles', a term which is perceived by patients as having malignant potential. A firm diagnosis is therefore reassuring.

Other differential diagnoses: epidermal naevi; dermatofibroma; melanoma; squamous cell carcinoma; basal cell carcinoma.

Conclusion and key points: apart from the morphology, the age of onset is a useful discriminator. Seborrhoeic keratoses occur infrequently below 30 years of age, whereas most naevi develop before this age. The typical crusted appearance of a seborrhoeic keratosis is rarely confused with naevi, but some naevi are remarkably warty and may cause diagnostic confusion; such naevi are usually quite deeply pigmented and have a soft surface. When they occur in younger patients, seborrhoeic keratoses are often less keratotic than in older individuals. In lesions without significant keratinization, there is typically a fairly uniform yellowish-brown colour and a greasy cobblestoned surface, and small white 'pearls' of keratin are usually visible.

Comparative features		
Disorder	**Naevus**	**Seborrhoeic keratosis**
Age	Present at any age but most develop before 30 yr	Mostly > 60 yr, uncommon below 40 yr
Sex	Either	
Family history	Non-specific	
Sites	Face, trunk, limbs	
Symptoms	None	Usually none. Keratotic lesions may be itchy.
Signs common to both	Discrete pigmented lesions	
Discriminatory signs	Smooth surface. If naevi have an elevated portion, this has a rubbery or fleshy feel. Some have increased numbers of hairs. Some have a warty surface and keratin plugs, and are more difficult to differentiate from seborrhoeic keratoses.	Rough or cobblestoned surface, often greasy texture, with keratin plugs (which may have a pseudofollicular appearance), and small yellowish-white keratin 'pearls'
Associated features	None	
Important tests	None	
Rationale for a firm diagnosis	Melanocytic naevi have a very small malignant potential. If removal is required to exclude malignancy, formal excision is the appropriate technique to use.	Seborrhoeic keratoses have no malignant potential, but can occasionally be confused with squamous cell carcinomas. In the few instances where removal is necessary, cryotherapy or curettage is usually the best treatment choice.

Further reading:
p. 12, pp. 46–50, p. 56, p. 128, p. 152, pp. 158–162.

References

Connors RC, Ackerman AB. Histologic pseudomalignancies of the skin. *Arch Dermatol* 1976; **112**:1767–80.

Stern RE, Boudreaux C, Arndt KA. Diagnostic accuracy and appropriateness of care for seborrhoeic keratoses. A pilot study of an approach to quality assurance for cutaneous surgery. *JAMA* 1991; **265**:74–77.

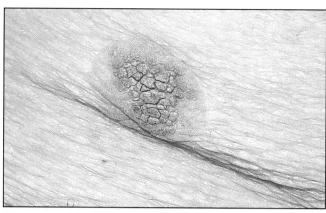

Figure 81.1 *Seborrhoeic keratosis, with a typical pale brown colour, 'cracked' appearance of surface, and flatter peripheral component.*

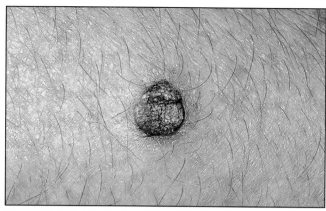

Figure 81.2 *'Irritated' seborrhoeic keratosis: lesions are darker, crusted and may be itchy. They may be confused with naevi or melanoma.*

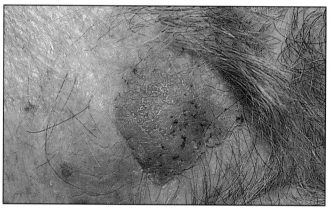

Figure 81.3 *Seborrhoeic keratosis: colour variation within these lesions is frequent. Note the greasy appearance of the surface.*

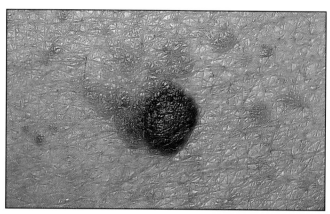

Figure 81.4 *Seborrhoeic keratosis, showing a darker lesion which may cause diagnostic problems. Note the flatter and paler portion which is more typical, and the 'pseudofollicles' in the darker portion.*

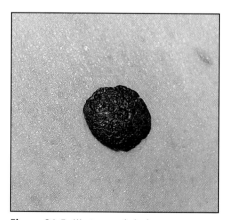

Figure 81.5 *Warty naevi: lesions are typically dark in colour, but have a soft surface. Note the absence here of a peripheral flatter portion (compare with Fig. 81.4).*

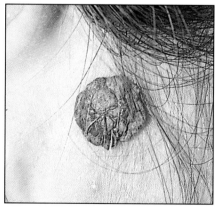

Figure 81.6 *Warty naevus on the temple. The history is important; this lesion had been present since birth.*

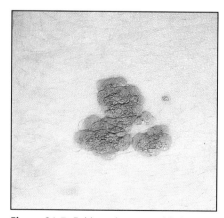

Figure 81.7 *Epidermal naevus: this is a form of birthmark which is typically keratotic and brown-coloured. However, it is usually linear or has a more irregular geographical outline compared with naevi or seborrhoeic keratoses.*

Common presenting feature: subcutaneous skin nodule.

Rationale for comparison: a correct diagnosis may influence the choice of operative technique in instances where treatment is required.

Other differential diagnoses: pilar cyst; true dermoid cyst (Fig. 25.4); skin appendage tumours (especially pilomatrixoma, apocrine hidrocystoma); keloids (especially rounded nodules on ears or at vaccination sites); rheumatoid nodules; neurofibromas.

Conclusion and key points: epidermoid cysts and lipomas are usually easy to differentiate on the basis of the following features. Epidermoid cysts usually occur on the head and neck, whereas lipomas are more common on the trunk and limbs. Epidermoid cysts are firm or hard, with a smooth surface and easy mobility under the skin, except for the tethering effect of a punctum. Pilar cysts on the scalp are less mobile and easy to define due to the thickness of the overlying skin; they do not have a punctum, and therefore rarely develop secondary infection. By contrast, lipomas are softer, more lobulated, less easy to define by palpation, and have no punctum. In tight areas of skin or in the case of deep lesions (e.g. frontalis-associated lipoma), the differential diagnosis may be difficult.

Comparative features		
Disorder	**Epidermoid cyst**	**Lipoma**
Age	Mostly young adult	Any
Sex	Either	
Family history	May be positive if multiple lesions; consider also steatocystoma multiplex in such cases	May be positive if lesions are multiple
Sites	Mainly head and neck, upper back	Mainly trunk and limbs
Symptoms	May be painful if rapidly enlarging, infected, or ruptured	Lipomas may be painful in some individuals. Such lesions are typically classified histologically as angiolipomas
Signs common to both	Subcutaneous swelling with overlying mobile skin	
Discriminatory signs	Epidermoid cysts have a smooth surface, hard or firm feel, and a white colour if visible through stretched skin. They have a punctum, through which cheesy white macerated keratin may be expressed. However, they may be more inflamed or feel tethered if there has been previous infection or rupture. Pilar cysts of scalp have a white or slightly blue colour, no punctum, and are thin-walled so may rupture during excision.	Lipomas have a softer and less well defined lobulated edge compared with cysts, and have a yellowish colour if they are visible through stretched skin. They have no punctum. Lipomas may become very large in some cases.
Associated features	None	
Important tests	None	
Treatment options (if required)	Excision can often be performed through a small incision; the entire sac and punctum should be removed to prevent recurrence. Ruptured lesions with persistent inflammation in the absence of secondary infection may respond to intralesional steroid injection.	Lipomas can generally be expressed through small skin incisions, with a pressure dressing to prevent haematoma in the 'dead space' post-operatively.

Further reading:
p. 48, p. 50, p. 152.

References
Belcher RW, *et al.* Multiple (subcutaneous) angiolipomas. *Arch Dermatol* 1974; **110**:583–5.

Salasche SJ, *et al.* Frontalis-associated lipoma of the forehead. *J Am Acad Dermatol* 1989;**20**:462–8.

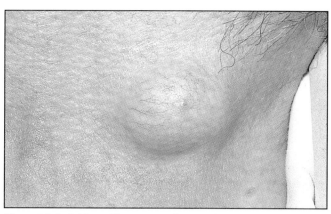

Figure 82.1 *Epidermoid cyst: note the stretched skin, steep-sided domed shape, and punctum.*

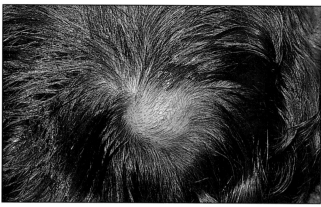

Figure 82.2 *Pilar cyst of scalp. The domed shape is typical. Lipomas rarely occur at this site. Note that the hair has been trimmed over the lesion. Alopecia is not a feature of skin over pilar cysts, though there may be some reduction in follicular density if the skin is significantly stretched.*

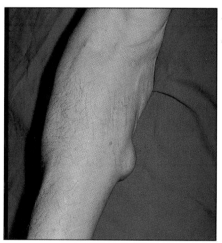

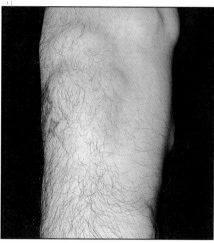

Figures 82.3 and 82.4 *Multiple lipomas: these have a shallower dome shape and softer texture. Multiple lesions may appear semiconfluent.*

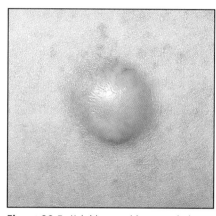

Figure 82.5 *Keloid scar: this may mimic a cyst, but is within the dermis. The skin is therefore fixed to the entire nodule rather than to an isolated punctum as occurs in epidermoid cysts.*

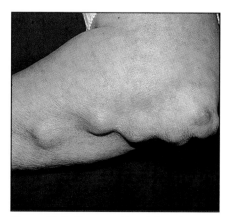

Figure 82.6 *Rheumatoid nodules: these are hard, and feel similar to cysts, but are characteristically located over bony prominences.*

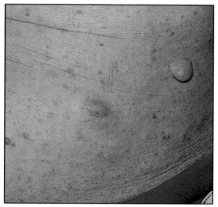

Figure 82.7 *Neurofibromas: these may be solitary or multiple. They are typically slightly pedunculated, soft in texture, and compressible through an underlying dermal defect. They may be confused with cysts or naevi.*

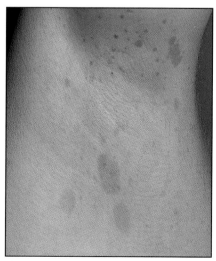

Figure 82.8 *Axillary freckling (Crowe's sign), a useful sign of neurofibromatosis.*

83 Multiple minute Campbell de Morgan spots v. purpura

Common presenting feature: punctate, blood-coloured lesions.

Rationale for comparison: multiple minute Campbell de Morgan spots are a common normal finding, which may be confused with purpura or vasculitis and therefore lead to extensive but unnecessary investigations.

Other differential diagnoses: angioma serpiginosum; hereditary haemorrhagic telangiectasia (p. 44); small vessel vasculitis (e.g. Henoch–Schönlein, drug-induced).

Conclusion and key points: multiple minute Campbell de Morgan spots are long-standing tiny angiomas but may suddenly be noticed by patients or doctors. Close examination reveals a vascular structure rather than the more blotchy or stellate pattern of extravasated blood; some larger and more typical Campbell de Morgan spots are usually present in patients with multiple small lesions. Distinction from extravasated blood can be difficult, as the small size of the minute Campbell de Morgan spots makes it difficult to blanch them without obscuring them from view.

Most causes of purpura do not have specific cutaneous features, but some causes of capillary leakage, such as vitamin C deficiency, may be easily clinically diagnosable. Due to the combined effects of vasodilatation and gravitational pressure, purpura is common within inflammatory dermatoses affecting the legs and does not require investigation unless out of proportion to the background eruption.

Comparative features		
Disorder	**Multiple minute Campbell de Morgan spots**	**Purpura**
Age	Usually apparent in young adult	Any
Sex	Either, probably female predominance	Either
Family history	Non-specific	
Sites	Most obvious on trunk and arms	Most apparent on legs
Symptoms	None	None due to the purpura itself
Signs common to both	Punctate blood-coloured lesions	
Discriminatory signs	Close-up examination reveals vascular structure.	Close-up examination reveals blotch or stellate morphology. Purpura may have a perifollicular distribution, especially in vitamin C deficiency.
Associated features	Some larger Campbell de Morgan spots also present	Larger purpuric or ecchymotic areas suggest haematological causes. In small vessel vasculitis, small purpuric lesions are often palpable, and there may be some larger crusted lesions. Systemic features, such as haematuria, may also be apparent in vasculitis. In scurvy, follicular keratoses, purpura, and 'corkscrew' hairs precede frank bleeding in muscles or from the gums.
Important tests	None	Haematological and coagulation screen, investigations for causes and consequences of systemic vasculitis

Further reading:
p. 44, p. 140, p. 158.

References
Colver GB, Kemmett D. Eruptive capillary haemangiomas. *Arch Dermatol* 1991; **127**:127–8.
Cox NH, Paterson WD. Angioma serpiginosum: a simulator of purpura. *Postgrad Med J* 1991; **67**:1065–6.

Piette WW. Primary systemic vasculitis. In: Sontheimer RD, Provost TT (eds). *Cutaneous manifestations of rheumatic diseases*. Williams & Wilkins, Baltimore, 1996:177–232.

Figure 83.1 *Multiple minute Campbell de Morgan spots: this is a distant view to demonstrate the density of lesions.*

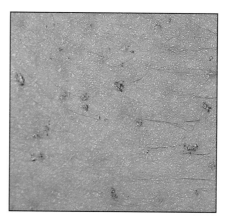

Figure 83.2 *Multiple minute Campbell de Morgan spots: a close-up view demonstrates that individual clusters of blood vessels can be identified.*

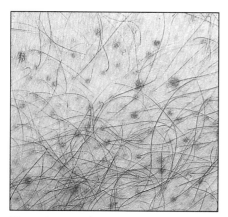

Figure 83.3 *Leukocytoclastic small vessel vasculitis: lesions have extravasated blood and are less sharply demarcated compared with the intact vessels in Fig. 83.2.*

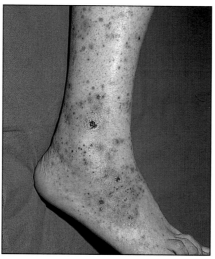

Figure 83.4 *Henoch–Schönlein purpura on the lower legs (a typical site) with some crusted lesions.*

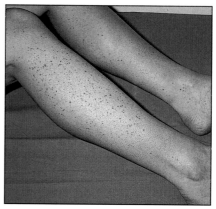

Figure 83.5 *Waldenstrom's hypergammaglobulinaemic purpura: this typically presents as episodic transient tiny areas of purpura on the legs in women. It has a benign course, and should not be confused with macroglobulinaemia.*

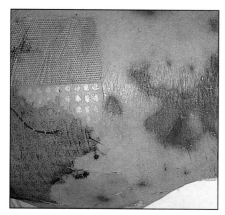

Figure 83.6 *Meningococcal vasculitis: tiny lesions may occur, but the stellate morphology shown here is characteristic.*

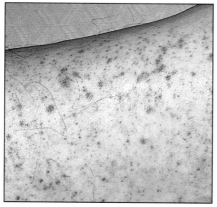

Figure 83.7 *Subacute bacterial endocarditis producing a non-specific pattern of small vessel vasculitis known as 'palpable purpura'.*

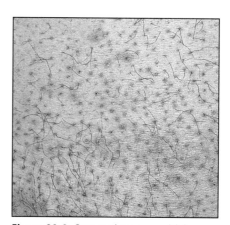

Figure 83.8 *Scurvy: there are multiple purpuric lesions with a typical perifollicular distribution.*

Common presenting feature: asymmetrical acute erythema (confluent or patches) with itch or pain.

Rationale for comparison: herpes zoster requires early treatment for this to have any benefit, but this stage of the eruption may be difficult to diagnose. It should be considered in the differential diagnosis of any unilateral acutely itchy or painful eruption, but may be asymptomatic.

Other differential diagnoses: are numerous and considered here in two groups. (1) Acute inflammatory conditions, e.g. eczemas; bacterial infections; herpes simplex infections (especially eczema herpeticum or herpes simplex at non-facial sites); and bullous eruptions, e.g. drug-induced photosensitivity. (2) Acute disorders with a linear or dermatomal pattern, especially phyto- or phytophoto-dermatitis (which may exhibit both linearity and blistering) and lichen striatus.

Conclusion and key points: although a direct comparison of two specific diseases is not being made here, this is an important topic because of the potential diagnostic difficulty and need for early therapy. Herpes zoster lesions often take a few days to develop dermatomal distribution, and may present as isolated plaques within a dermatome. This is particularly likely in early lesions, but some never progress beyond this pattern. The diagnosis should be considered in any acute unilateral eruption, especially with the clue of dermatomal symptoms, and especially if there are risk factors (elderly, immunosuppressed). Blisters are typically larger and less monomorphic than in herpes simplex. Diagnostic confusion may also occur when herpes zoster is associated with multiple disseminated lesions (as in chickenpox); this occurs in about 15% of patients.

Comparative features		
Disorder	**Herpes zoster**	**Examples of other acute inflammatory eruptions**
Age	The incidence increases with age	Erysipelas of face—middle age and elderly Herpes simplex—young adult Lichen striatus—child Plant contact—any
Sex	Either	
Family history	Herpes zoster occasionally occurs as clusters or at times when chickenpox is frequent in the community, presumably by immunological reactivation of latent virus. Non-immune contacts can catch chickenpox from patients with herpes zoster.	Depends on cause. Mostly non-specific
Sites	Unilateral, dermatomal (may affect only part of the dermatome, especially in early lesions). Distribution is about 15% trigeminal (increases with age), 20% cervical, 50% trunk, 15% lumbosacral.	Erysipelas—mid-facial (Figs 21.1, 21.2), lower leg Herpes simplex—face, genital/buttock/thigh Lichen striatus—limb Plant contact—mainly arms
Symptoms	Dermatomal pain or itch (may precede visible skin eruption)	Local pain or itch (lichen striatus is usually asymptomatic)
Signs common to both	Discrete erythematous plaque(s) +/- vesiculation or bullae	
Discriminatory signs	Unilateral, extends within a single dermatome (may be 2 or 3 adjacent dermatomes in sacral area). Palatal involvement may be a useful discriminator if present in patients with maxillary zoster. Lesions evolve from vesicle to pustule to crust.	Erysipelas—usually becomes rapidly symmetrical and is associated with significant pyrexia (as is lower leg cellulitis, which is unilateral but not dermatomal). Herpes simplex—smaller blisters and remains localized. Lichen striatus—narrower band, not dermatomal, not painful. Plant contact—more streaky, not dermatomal, leaves residual brown pigmentation
Associated features	May be some scattered vesicles resembling chickenpox (if >20, consider immune status) or underlying malignancy. May be motor involvement, ocular involvement if facial, regional lymphadenopathy	Depends on cause
Important tests	Diagnose by Tzank smear, culture, ELISA, electron microscopy, serology	Dictated by likely causes

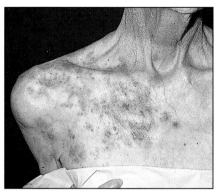

Figure 84.1 *Herpes zoster with typical midline demarcation. This eruption occurred in a patient having chemotherapy. It caused a diagnostic problem as it was confined to the tip of the shoulder for the first 24 hours.*

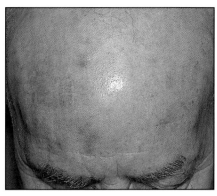

Figure 84.2 *Herpes zoster on the forehead, with unilateral but patchy distribution. It was not obviously dermatomal or with a midline cut-off. Acute rosacea was part of the differential diagnosis.*

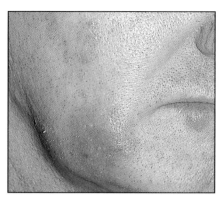

Figure 84.3 *Herpes zoster with unilateral distribution, but individually discrete lesions.*

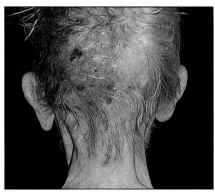

Figure 84.4 *Herpes zoster in C2 dermatome, effecting only the scalp, with typical midline cut-off. The degree of crusting on the scalp may cause diagnostic problems.*

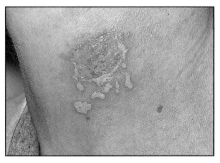

Figure 84.5 *Herpes simplex on the neck, with associated dysphagia and swelling of soft tissues. The referral diagnosis was cellulitis, and the symptoms suggested the possibility of herpes zoster, but the grouped small vesicles were typical of herpes simplex.*

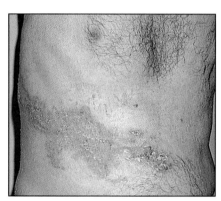

Figure 84.6 *Herpes zoster of the trunk, with typical linear dermatomal pattern.*

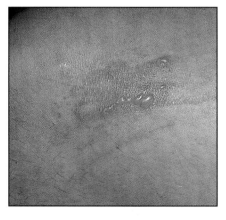

Figure 84.7 *Phytophoto-dermatitis: this is typically caused by the hogweed family of hedgerow plants. This exhibits both linearity and blistering with acute pain.*

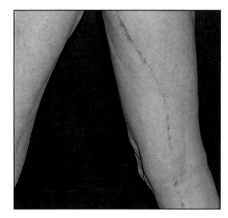

Figure 84.8 *Lichen striatus: an acute-onset, but usually asymptomatic, eruption with linear distribution along a limb. The affected band of skin is too narrow to be compatible with herpes zoster, and the distribution is not dermatomal.*

Further reading:
p. 42.

References
Huff JC. Herpes zoster. *Curr Prob Dermatol* 1988; **1**:8–40.
Izumi AK, Edwards J. Herpes zoster with neurogenic bladder dysfunction. *Arch Dermatol* 1974; **109**:692–4.

Nahass GT, *et al*. The clinical spectrum from classic varicella zoster to zoster sine herpete: the missing link. *Arch Dermatol* 1992; **128**:1278–9.
Palmer SR, *et al*. An outbreak of shingles? *Lancet* 1985; **ii**:1108–11.

85 Chronic paronychia v. dermatophyte (tinea) infection

Common presenting feature: nailplate dystrophy.

Rationale for comparison: different causes, and usually different treatments.

Other differential diagnoses: traumatic dystrophies, (habit tic of fingernails, bilateral hallux nail dystrophy, p. 172, Fig. 86.1); ingrown nail; ischaemic nail; idiopathic and other causes of onycholysis; congenital nail dystrophies in children; psoriatic nail (p. 174, Fig. 88.5); periungual inflammation causing secondary nail-plate damage (eczemas, psoriasis, connective tissue disorders); squamous cell carcinoma (Fig. 89.2).

Conclusion and key points: chronic paronychia, or inflammation of the soft tissue of the nailfold, is usually due to *Candida* infection, but is not a feature of dermatophyte fungal infection. It is manifest as erythema and swelling ('bolstering') of the nailfold, with loss of the cuticle and sometimes discharge from the nailfold. It may occur as a consequence of abnormal nails distorting the nailfold, or without primary nailplate damage; it may also cause nail surface ridges and distortion. Dermatophyte nail infection is most commonly subungual, with nailplate thickening and onycholysis but without nailfold changes. In children, congenital dystrophies, trauma and paronychia are all much more common than tinea infection. Chronic paronychia should usually be treated by topical applications to the nailfold, while tinea of the nail (unless mild) requires systemic treatment. Although itraconazole will kill both yeasts and dermatophytes, systemic griseofulvin and terbinafine will not eradicate yeasts in chronic paronychia. Confirmation of a dermatophyte should always be obtained by culture of nail clippings, before introducing systemic therapy, as other commensal organisms are likely to be resistant to therapy (e.g. *Scopulariopsis brevicaulis*).

Comparative features		
Disorder	**Chronic paronychia**	**Dermatophyte (tinea) infection of nail**
Age	Any. In children, the commonest site is the thumb due to sucking.	Any, but rare in children
Sex	Either	
Family history	Non-specific	Sometimes infection of nails, or associated tinea pedis, is present in other family members.
Sites	Nailfold, usually one or more fingernails	Subungual nailplate thickening, most frequently of the toenails. In the commonest type, infection spreads from distal or lateral aspects towards the proximal nail (Fig. 85.5).
Symptoms	Variable pain, tenderness, intermittent discharge	Usually none but may be pressure effects due to thickened nail
Signs common to both	Nail plate dystrophy	
Discriminatory signs	Presence of nailfold thickening and loss of cuticle (i.e. paronychia). Secondary nailplate damage is generally manifest as horizontal ridges. This starts adjacent to the site of the main nailfold abnormality, hence initial distortion is usually apparent proximally. Thickening of the entire nailplate may occur as a late feature.	Absence of paronychia. Other positive features are subungual hyperkeratosis, onycholysis, discoloration (yellow, white or brown) seen through the nailplate. A less common form of dermatophyte infection (superficial white onychomycosis) affects the surface of the nailplate which is crumbly. Proximal subungual onychomycosis is a rarer variant which produces white colour under the nail and spreads distally from the nailfold.
Associated features	None	Frequently, tinea pedis
Important tests	Scrape from under nailfold for culture (yeasts and bacteria)	Clippings from nail for microscopy and mycology culture (Fig. 55.7)
Predisposing factors	Wet work (by housewives, publicans, domestic cleaners, etc.), damage to cuticles by manicuring, inflammatory dermatoses around nailfolds	Presence of cutaneous tinea (pp. 58, 62, 110) Other nail dystrophies

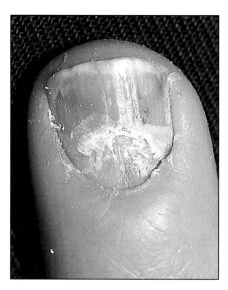

Figure 85.1 *Chronic paronychia with candidal infection of the proximal nail-fold, producing a 'bolstered' appearance.*

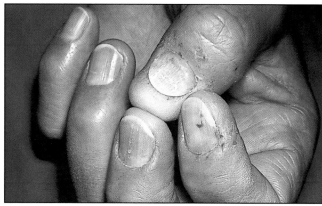

Figure 85.2 *Chronic paronychia of several nails. This may be traumatic, especially in individuals who pick at the area, but also occurs as a consequence of inflammatory dermatoses in the periungual area, such as eczemas.*

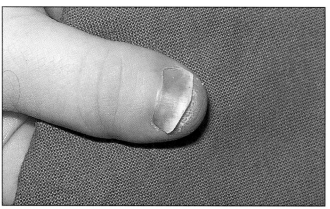

Figure 85.3 *Nail dystrophy and mild chronic paronychia in a child due to thumb-sucking.*

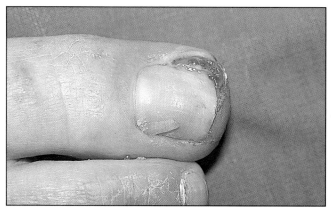

Figure 85.4 *Ingrowing toenail: this may be confused with fungal infections.*

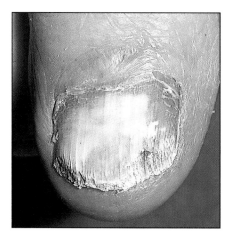

Figure 85.5 *Dermatophyte infection of a toenail: this is a common pattern known as distal and lateral subungual onychomycosis. Note the colour changes and subungual hyperkeratosis, but lack of damage to the proximal nail-fold.*

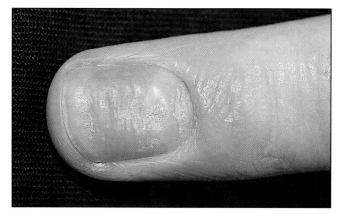

Figure 85.6 *Chronic paronychia with nail-plate surface damage due to atopic dermatitis.*

Further reading:
p. 62, p. 68, p. 110, p. 120, pp. 172–176.

References
Denning DW, *et al*. Fungal nail disease: a guide to good practice. *BMJ* 1995; **311**:1277–81.
Hay RJ. Onychomycosis. Agents of choice. *Dermatol Clinics* 1993; **11**:161–9.

Roberts DT. Oral therapeutic agents in fungal nail disease. *J Am Acad Dermatol* 1994; **31**:578–91.
Shwayder T. Pediatric nail disorders. *Semin Dermatol* 1995; **14**:21–6.

86 Traumatic toenail dystrophy v. tinea of toenails

Common presenting feature: thickened discoloured hallux (and occasionally other) toenails.

Rationale for comparison: it is not widely recognized that recurrent and often minor trauma, such as that due to footwear, causes a nail dystrophy. Like tinea infections of feet and nails, traumatic dystrophy is common in young men, probably due to sporting activities. There is therefore potential for the two diagnoses to be confused, but their treatments are entirely different.

Other differential diagnoses: congenital malalignment of toenails; pincer nails; subungual haematoma without dystrophy (Fig. 90.4); ingrowing toenail (Fig. 85.4); subungual exostosis (Fig. 89.7); subungual melanoma (p. 180).

Conclusion and key points: symmetrical dystrophy of hallux nails in young men (or sometimes the nail of the second toe), especially without other nail abnormalities, is more likely to be due to repetitive minor trauma than to fungal infection. Traumatic nail dystrophy may occur due to one, or a combination, of the following: shoes that are too small; playing football; regular running. Treatment consists of attention to footwear, rather than medication. A solitary nail dystrophy in a young adult may be due to subungual exostosis (p. 178, Fig. 89.7) and is an indication for X-ray radiography. Traumatic dystrophies of fingernails are not included in the specific comparison in this section, but are illustrated as they are also often confused with fungal infections.

Comparative features		
Disorder	**Traumatic nail dystrophy**	**Tinea of toenail**
Age	Mainly young adult (often symmetrical)	Adult
Sex	Usually male if symmetrical, either sex if discrete injury	Either
Family history	Negative	Non-specific
Sites	Usually hallux nails but may affect the second toe if this is the longest toe. An isolated discrete injury may affect any nail.	Any nail
Symptoms	Usually none unless there has been a recent injury	Usually none unless gross thickening
Signs common to both	Thickened discoloured toenail	
Discriminatory signs	May be subungual haematoma (p. 180). Most confusion is with minor repetetive injury, usually causing symmetrical hallux nail dystrophy. Splinter haemorrhages are a frequent feature.	Usually asymmetrical. Discoloration often includes shades of white or yellow. Crumbly undersurface of nail plate present, except in superficial white onychomycosis in which case the external surface of the nailplate is affected
Associated features	None are helpful. Traumatic nail dystrophy is typically a problem of young men who play football; tinea pedis is therefore also common.	Tinea at other parts of foot is frequent but does not in itself prove that the nail dystrophy is fungal in origin.
Important tests	None	Clip nail for microscopy and mycology culture.

Further reading:
p. 62, p. 68, p. 110, p. 120, p. 170, pp. 174–178.

References
Daniel CR III. The diagnosis of nail fungal infection. *Arch Dermatol* 1991; **127**:1566–7.

Denning DW, *et al.* Fungal nail disease: a guide to good practice. *BMJ* 1995; **311**:1277–81.
Zaias N. Onychomycosis. *Arch Dermatol* 1972; **105**:263–74.

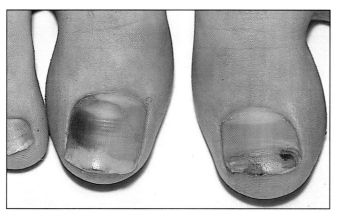

Figure 86.1 *Symmetrical hallux subungual discoloration due to repetitive trauma.*

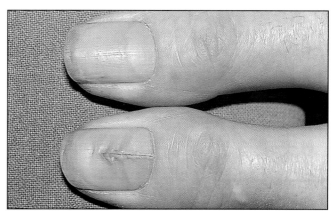

Figure 86.2 *Median canaliform dystrophy of fingernails, demonstrating the typical fir-tree pattern. This nail dystrophy may also be confused with fungal infection.*

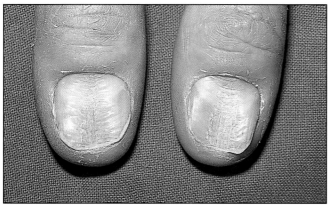

Figure 86.3 *Tic dystrophy of fingernails: this is caused by a habit of picking at the nails and is frequently confused with fungal infection.*

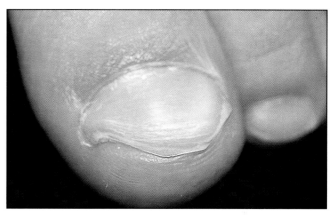

Figure 86.4 *Koilonychia of a toenail: this is a common normal finding in young children and is not due to fungal infection or nutritional deficiency.*

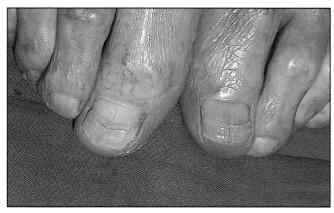

Figure 86.5 *Beau's lines, with incipient nail shedding (onychomadesis) following hospital admission for bullous pemphigoid and streptococcal cellulitis.*

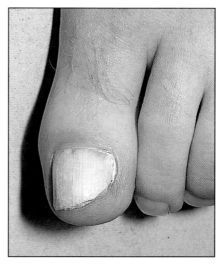

Figure 86.6
Aspergillus *infection of nail: this is impossible to distinguish from a dermatophyte infection on clinical grounds, and demonstrates the importance of obtaining results of mycology samples, rather than starting 'blind' treatment.*

87 Psoriasis v. eczema

Common presenting feature: nail dystrophy associated with inflammatory skin disease.

Rationale for comparison: the nail changes may be a useful feature to distinguish between the two skin disorders when there is diagnostic uncertainty.

Other differential diagnoses: fungal nail dystrophy (p. 170): paronychia (p. 170); other inflammatory dermatoses with nail changes (e.g. pityriasis rubra pilaris, lichen planus, Darier's disease); other causes of nail pitting or surface changes (e.g. trachyonychia).

Conclusion and key points: psoriasis of the nails tends to have a more specific appearance than nail dystrophy related to eczema. The psoriatic features may be sufficiently characteristic to allow psoriasis of nails to be diagnosed in patients who have nail involvement without skin lesions elsewhere. Pitting is neater in psoriasis compared with the ridged and rippled appearance in eczema. Onycholysis, proximal nail-bed reddish-brown discoloration (salmon patches, or oil-drop lesions), subungual hyperkeratosis and splinter haemorrhages are all features of psoriasis of nails. Subungual pustules and nail destruction are rare. Patients with eczema may have nail changes due to scratching and rubbing (polished nails, bevelled free edge of nails), as well as pitting and transverse ridging related to eczema of the nailfolds.

Comparative features

Disorder	Psoriasis (nail)	Eczema (nail)
Age	Any	
Sex	Either	
Family history	Often positive	
Sites	Any nail	
Symptoms	Usually none. May be pressure effects or difficulty cutting thick hyperkeratotic nail; sharp edges may catch on clothing. Subungual pustules may be painful, periungual psoriasis may be itchy or painful.	None, or itch due to periungual eczema
Signs common to both	Dystrophic nail plate, pitting of nails, splinter haemorrhages, +/- periungual rash and paronychia	
Discriminatory signs	Pitting is typically profuse and regular. Onycholysis has pink or yellowish coloured proximal border; this subungual 'salmon–patch' or 'oil–drop' appearance is typical of psoriasis. Subungual hyperkeratosis is more prominent than in eczema. Pustules and destruction of the nail plate are a feature of psoriasis variants.	Pitting is more irregular and rippled in appearance. Other nail changes due to scratching skin lesions are most frequent in eczemas but not specific to this cause; they include a polished appearance of the nail plate and concave bevelling of the free edge of the nail.
Associated features	Psoriatic nail changes may occur in isolation, but are more common in association with psoriasis at typical sites, e.g. elbows, knees, scalp.	Eczematous nail changes are uncommon in the absence of current (or recent) dermatitis of hands, and there may be eczema at other body sites. Chronic paronychia (p. 170) is usually present.
Important tests	Exclude fungal infection by mycology of nail clippings if clinically indicated, but be aware that saprophytic fungi and some *Candida* species may colonize the space created by onycholysis. Visualizing fungal elements does not prove that they are pathogenic in situations where there is existing nail dystrophy.	Usually none specific to the nail. Eczema confined to fingertips may have an allergic cause and patch testing is required.

Further reading:
p. 2, pp. 58–68, p. 76, p. 82, p. 84, p. 102, p. 110, p. 118, p. 170, p. 172, p. 176.

References
Baran R, Dawber RPR. The nail in dermatological disease. In: Baran R, Dawber RPR (eds). *Diseases of the nails and their management*, 2nd edn. Blackwell Scientific Publishers, Oxford, 1994:135–73.

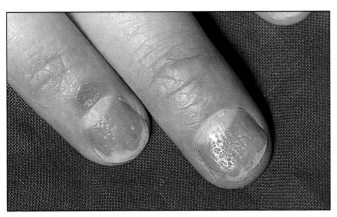

Figure 87.1 *Psoriasis: the typical regular pattern of pitting resembles the surface of a thimble.*

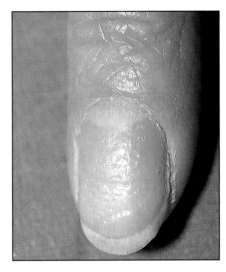

Figure 87.2
Eczema of nailfold with nail dystrophy demonstrating a less specific 'rippled' pattern of transverse ridges.

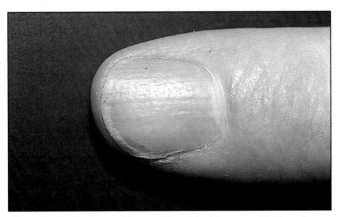

Figure 87.3 *Trachyonychia, associated in this case with alopecia areata. This is a finer pattern of pitting which may produce a rough 'sand-papered' appearance of the nailplate.*

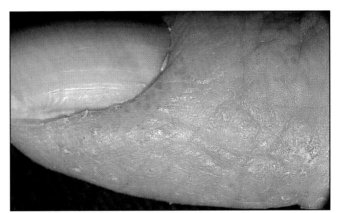

Figure 87.4 *Vesicles adjacent to the nail in a patient with nail dystrophy due to eczema.*

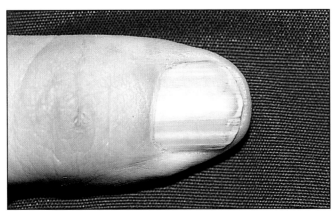

Figure 87.5 *Darier's disease with typical white discoloration, longitudinal splitting of the nail, and notching of the free edge of the nailplate.*

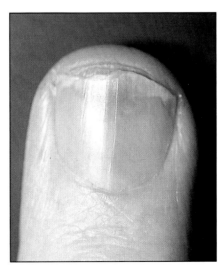

Figure 87.6
Psoriasis, showing onycholysis, subungual hyperkeratosis, and greasy pinkish subungual discoloration (oil drop sign).

88 Psoriasis v. dermatophyte (tinea) infection

Common presenting feature: one or several dystrophic nails.

Rationale for comparison: commonly confused diagnostically which may lead to unnecessary antifungal therapy.

Other differential diagnoses: paronychia with secondary nail dystrophy (p. 170); eczemas (p. 174); ischaemia; yellow nail syndrome; onychogryphosis; other inflammatory dermatoses; trachyonychia.

Conclusion and key points: the presence of psoriasis does not preclude fungal infection, and may encourage it, but a firm distinction between these disorders can often be made on morphological grounds. It is important to take appropriate samples for microscopy and mycological cultures where doubt exists. Note that saprophytic fungi (e.g. *Scopulariopsis brevicaulis*) and some *Candida* spp. (e.g. *C. parapsilosis*) may colonize the space created by onycholysis. Visualizing fungal elements does not prove that they are pathogenic in situations where there is existing nail dystrophy. Patients who have been treated with long and ineffective courses of antifungal therapy despite negative cultures are common dermatology referrals; many have a psoriatic nail dystrophy.

Comparative features		
Disorder	**Psoriasis (nail)**	**Tinea (nail)**
Age	Any	Any, but uncommon in children
Sex	Either	
Family history	Often positive	Non-specific
Sites	Any nail (usually multiple), fingers or toes	Any nail. Frequently solitary, especially in the case of fingernails, or asymmetrical if multiple nails are affected. If fingernails are affected, consider *Candida* as well as dermatophyte fungal infection. If many fingernails are affected, the fungi present may be saprophytes colonizing previously dystrophic nails, rather than being the cause of the dystrophy.
Symptoms	None, or pressure effect due to hyperkeratosis	
Signs common to both	Dystrophic nail with prominent subungual hyperkeratosis	
Discriminatory signs	Pitting of the nailplate. Subungual reddish-brown discoloration proximal to any area of onycholysis, known as the 'salmon–patch' or 'oil–drop' sign (Fig. 87.6). The specific psoriatic signs are generally more definite in fingernails compared with toenails.	None that is specific in the commonest types of tinea unguium (distal/lateral subungual onychomycosis). Superficial white onychomycosis and proximal subungual onychomycosis are more recognizable.
Associated features	Psoriasis at other sites	Tinea pedis
Important tests	None if the appearances are typical, but send samples for microscopy and mycological culture if there is uncertainty	Obtain results of microscopy and mycological culture prior to use of systemic therapy. This test not only confirms the presence of fungi to justify the treatment, but also distinguishes between dermatophytes, saprophytes and *Candida* species.

Further reading:
p. 2, pp. 58–64, p. 82, p. 84, p. 102, p. 110, p. 120, pp. 170–174.

References
Cohen PR, Scher RK. Geriatric nail disorders: diagnosis and treatment. *J Am Acad Dermatol* 1992; **26**:521–31.

Samman PD, Strickland B. Abnormalities of the fingernails associated with impaired peripheral blood supply. *Br J Dermatol* 1962; **74**:65–8.

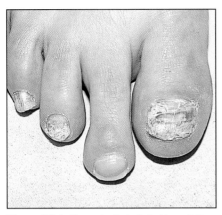

Figure 88.1 *Dermatophyte infection of the nail, with typical colour changes and nail-plate damage.*

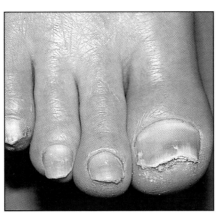

Figure 88.2 *Ischaemic nail changes: these may resemble tinea unguium.*

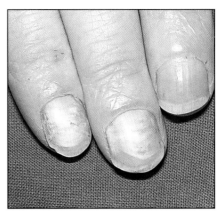

Figure 88.3 *Subungual onychomycosis due to* Trichophyton rubrum *producing white areas under the nailplate.*

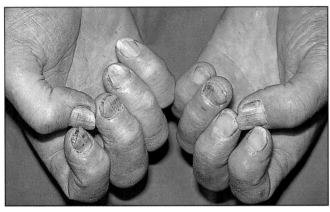

Figure 88.4 *Nail dystrophy of several fingernails: this was probably traumatic in origin due to manual work and frequent mechanical cleaning of subungual debris. Mycology demonstrated a saprophytic organism,* Scopulariopsis brevicaulis.

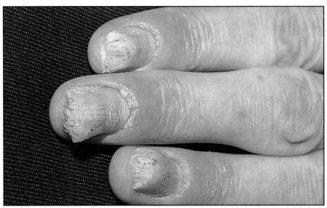

Figure 88.5 *Psoriatic nail dystrophy affecting several nails, with marked subungual hyperkeratosis. Involvement of many nails is uncommon in primary dermatophyte fingernail infections (less uncommon in toenails), and should suggest that a fungal cause is doubtful.*

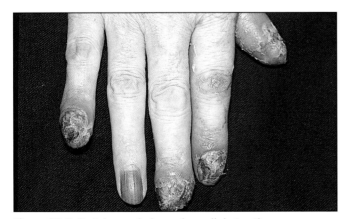

Figure 88.6 *Pustular psoriasis causing nail destruction.*

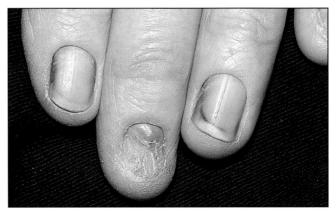

Figure 88.7 *Yellow nail syndrome: this disorder is associated with chronic lung sepsis and with lymphoedema. Nails are thickened and yellow, with increased transverse and longitudinal curvature. They grow very slowly, and may be shed, as in this case. There is no change in the surface of the nail and no crumbly subungual hyperkeratosis occurs.*

177

89 Periungual wart v. other periungual nodules

Common presenting feature: crusted, sometimes painful, nodule in the region of the nail; nail dystrophy can also occur. Examples of direct comparisons with warts considered here are subungual exostosis and digital myxoid cyst.

Rationale for comparison: there are several relatively common conditions arising in the vicinity of the nail which may be confused with warts but which require totally different therapies.

Other differential diagnoses: subungual exostosis (most commonly under a toenail); myxoid cyst (most commonly the dorsal aspect of the finger proximal to the nail); heloma (corn); periungual fibroma; glomus tumour; squamous cell carcinoma; malignant melanoma.

Conclusion and key points: warts in the region of the nail are much more common on fingers than toes, are usually multiple, and are more commonly periungual than subungual. Subungual exostoses are not uncommon, usually occurring in teenagers and young adults, and usually affect a single toenail (though they can occur under a fingernail). Radiological examination will confirm an exostosis, which should be treated by surgical removal. Digital myxoid (mucous) cysts occur on the dorsal aspect of the distal phalanx of the finger. They may extrude jelly-like material and may cause indentation or grooving of the nailplate. Glomus tumours are exquisitely painful subungual nodules which may be visibly red through the nail.

Comparative features		
Disorder	**Periungual wart**	**Other periungual nodules: subungual exostosis and digital myxoid cyst**
Age	Mostly teenagers and young adults	Exostosis: mostly teenagers and young adults Myxoid cyst: adults, mostly middle-aged
Sex	Either	
Family history	Non-specific	
Sites	Warts around the nail are most likely on fingers. They usually affect the proximal and lateral nailfolds, dorsal distal phalanx, or fingertip. Occasionally, they may be subungual (but rarely without other sites also being affected).	Exostosis: subungual, usually affecting a solitary toe but can occur under fingernails Myxoid cyst: dorsal aspect of distal phalanx, usually fingers
Symptoms	None or pain	
Signs common to both	Periungual nodules, with associated nail dystrophy	
Discriminatory signs	Usually have an obviously verrucous surface. Frequently multiple. Associated nail dystrophy is usually a shallow groove or indentation of the dorsal aspect of the nailplate, but subungual warts may cause distal elevation of the nail.	Exostosis: solitary subungual lesions. The surface is smoother than in a wart, but may be crusted. Distal nail elevation occurs. Myxoid cyst: smooth-surfaced dome-shaped nodule with a clear jelly-like fluid content, which may discharge. If there is associated nail dystrophy, the groove is similar to that caused by proximal nailfold warts.
Associated features	None	Exostosis: none Myxoid cyst: osteoarthritis of the distal interphalangeal joint, and Heberden's nodes
Important tests	None	Exostosis: X-ray radiiography
Treatment	None, salicylic acid gels, cryotherapy	Exostosis: partial or total nail avulsion and removal of the exostosis Myxoid cyst: none, intralesional steroid, cryotherapy (prolonged freeze times), surgical

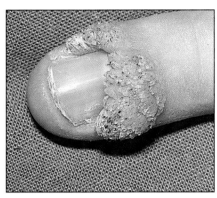

Figure 89.1 *Typical periungual wart note the verrucous surface and indented groove in the surface of the nailplate.*

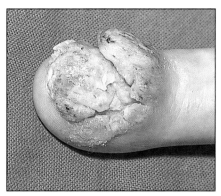

Figure 89.2 *Squamous cell carcinoma of the finger. This has a warty appearance, but note the destruction of the nail (sse also Fig. 35.7).*

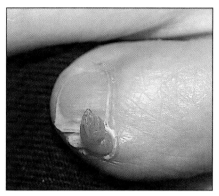

Figure 89.3 *Periungual fibroma. These may be multiple in tuberous sclerosis (p. 34), but also occur as sporadic solitary lesions.*

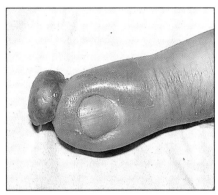

Figure 89.4 *Pyogenic granuloma of the fingertip. These lesions are typically very vascular and bleed easily, but patients may erroneously treat them with proprietary wart preparations.*

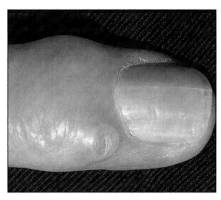

Figure 89.5 *Digital myxoid cyst found on the dorsum of the distal phalanx. These also cause a groove in the nailplate.*

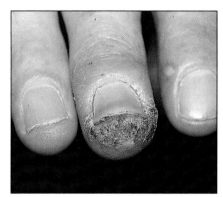

Figure 89.6 *Subungual warts. These are a refractory pattern and may cause diagnostic confusion. However, as in this case, there is usually a periungual wart present in the same or other fingernails.*

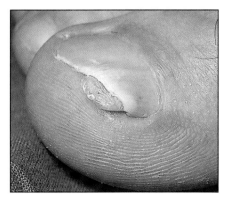

Figure 89.7
Subungual exostosis of a toenail. This presents as a painful crusted nodule under the nail.

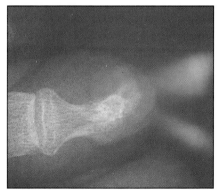

Figure 89.8
Subungual exostosis: shown here in a patient different from that of Fig. 89.7, demonstrating the radiological appearance which confirms the diagnosis.

Further reading
p. 72.

References
Baran R, *et al*. A text atlas of nail disorders. *Diagnosis and treatment*. Martin Dunitz, London, 1996:98–114.

Bart RS, *et al*. Acquired digital fibrokeratoma. *Arch Dermatol* 1968; **97**: 120–9.

de Berker DAR, *et al*. Micrographic surgery for subungual squamous cell carcinoma. *Br J Plast Surg* 1996; **49**:414–19.

Kato H, *et al*. Subungual exostosis: clinicopathological and ultrastructural studies of 3 cases. *Clin Exp Dermatol* 1990; **15**:429–32.

Common presenting feature: subungual pigmentation.

Rationale for comparison: unless particularly painful, the only treatment for a subungual haematoma is reassurance with no intervention being required. Subungual melanoma is potentially lethal and is usually treated by amputation.

Other differential diagnoses: other subungual tumours (squamous cell carcinoma, glomus tumour, naevus); other causes of longitudinal melanonychia and nail pigmentation (see Table).

Conclusion and key points: subungual pigmentation is a common cause of urgent referral; the vast majority of such patients have typical subungual haematoma. Remarkably, many patients are unaware of any specific trauma and uncertain of the duration of colour change, which is presumably due to damage from shoes. In some cases, when damage is distal or where sufficient time has elapsed, the damaged area is distal to the cuticle, producing a transverse, convex, curved, proximal border characteristic of haematoma. A wavy and divergent lateral border, associated splinter haemorrhages, or damage to adjacent nails, all support a diagnosis of haematoma. An obvious red colour is usually due to recent bleeding, but can occur in melanoma. If pigment extends to the free edge of the nail, it can be visualized as old clot adherent to the underneath of the nailplate in haematomas, whereas staining of the nailplate without visible clot occurs in cases of melanoma. Pigmentation of the skin distal to the nail is characteristic of melanoma, as is Hutchinson's sign (pigmentation of the nailfold), though the latter can be confusing if pigment is visible through this thin area of skin (pseudo-Hutchinson's sign). Associated nail damage, in the absence of a history of significant trauma, must be assumed to be due to melanoma.

Comparative features		
Disorder	**Subungual melanoma**	**Subungual haematoma**
Age	Usually middle-aged and elderly	Any, but occurrence in the absence of identifiable trauma falls into the same age-group as for melanoma
Sex	Either	Either, male predominance
Family history	Non-specific	
Sites	Usually thumb or hallux	Any digit; typically hallux in cases without definite history of trauma
Symptoms	Usually none	Usually painful, but a significant minority of cases are asymptomatic
Signs common to both	Subungual dark/black pigmentation	
Discriminatory signs	Pigmentation extending onto skin distal to the nail, or onto the proximal or lateral nailfold (Hutchinson's sign). Typically there is a uniform dark-brown pigment band known as longitudinal melanonychia: this is usually but not always due to melanocytic causes, and includes benign causes as well as melanoma (see Table). Nailplate destruction or damage without definite trauma is suggestive of melanoma.	In most cases, haematoma is distal to the proximal nailfold and has a sharply demarcated curved proximal limit. The lateral margins are wavy and divergent. Clot is visible at the free edge of the nail, adherent to the undersurface of the nail plate. Associated splinter haemorrhages may occur in the same or adjacent nails.
Associated features	This type of melanoma often presents at a late stage, so there may be regional lymphadenopathy.	May affect multiple nails (especially bilateral hallux involvement)
Important tests	Periungual melanoma is usually treated by amputation. Therefore, an initial incisional biopsy from the matrix origin of the pigmented band is usually performed to confirm the diagnosis.	Usually none. Confirmation of iron in material adherent to undersurface of nail (biochemical or with histological stains) supports haematoma. Careful measurement and documentation repeated after a month are useful methods to confirm that the haematoma is growing out distally. In some cases, however, a biopsy or partial/complete nail avulsion may be necessary.

Causes of longitudinal melanonychia	
Idiopathic	Normal feature in black skin (usually multiple), Laugier–Hunziker syndrome (with oral pigmentation)
Benign tumours	Naevi, lentigo
Malignant tumours	Melanoma, basal cell carcinoma, Bowen's disease
Infections	Fungi, *Pseudomonas*, *Aspergillus* (none of these usually longitudinal)
Systemic	Addison's disease, malnutrition, drugs, AIDS

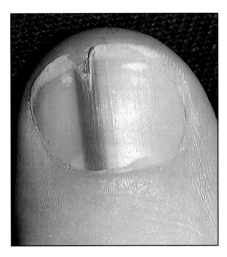

Figure 90.1
Pigmented nail streak due to a biopsy-proven simple lentigo. Note the linearity of the pigment and absence of nailfold pigmentation. In this case there was notching of the distal nailplate.

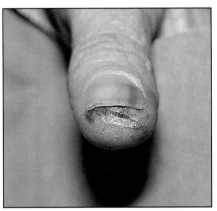

Figure 90.2 *Acral melanoma: pigmentation under the nail, spreading onto the tip of the digit.*

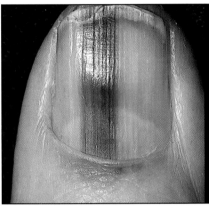

Figure 90.3 *Melanoma, showing a linear pigment band but with associated lateral spread along the proximal nailfold (Hutchinson's sign).*

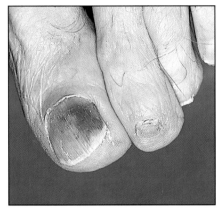

Figure 90.4 *Subungual haematoma. This is common on the hallux and has a blue colour. Note also the smaller subungual bruise under the adjacent second nail.*

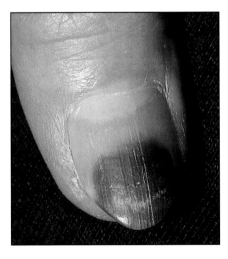

Figure 90.5
Pseudomonas *colonizing an area of onycholysis. This infection, and* Aspergillus *infection under the nail, typically produce dark pigmentation, which may be confused with melanoma.*

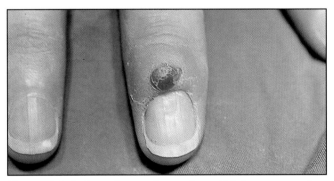

Figure 90.6 *Periungual pyogenic granuloma. This is a common site for this type of angioma in young patients. Amelanotic melanoma should be considered in older individuals.*

Further reading
p. 158, p. 160, p. 178.

References
Baran R, Kechijian P. Hutchinson's sign: a reappraisal. *J Am Acad Dermatol* 1996; **34**:87–90.

Baran R, Kechijian P. Longitudinal melanonychia (melanonychia striata): diagnosis and management. *J Am Acad Dermatol* 1989; **21**:1165–75.

Index

Index

Index